ft f   iners

Multi-sport
Training
for Fitness

Other titles in the Fitness Trainers series

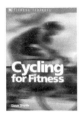

Cycling for Fitness
Dave Smith
ISBN 0-7136-5140-7
£13.99

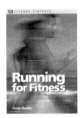

Interval Training for Fitness
Joseph Nitti and Kimberlie Nitti
ISBN 0-7136-6382-0
£13.99

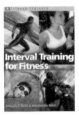

Running for Fitness
Owen Barder
ISBN 0-7136-5139-3
£13.99

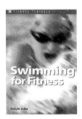

Swimming for Fitness
Kelvin Juba
ISBN 0-7136-5825-8
£13.99

ft Fitness Trainers

Multi-sport
Training
for Fitness

Fiona Hayes

A & C Black • London

Published in 2004 by
A & C Black Publishers Ltd
37 Soho Square, London W1D 3QZ
www.acblack.com

ISBN 0 7136 6654 4

A CIP catalogue record for this book is available from the British Library.

Note: Whilst every effort has been made to ensure that the content of this book is as technically accurate and as sound as possible, neither the authors nor the publishers can accept any responsibility for any injury or loss sustained as a result of the use of this material.

Acknowledgements
Cover photographs © Imagestate

Typeset in 10/12pt Minion Display

Printed and bound in Great Britain by Biddles, King's Lynn

Contents

I Introduction

II How to get started

III Multi-sport training programmes

IV Useful resources

Part I
Introduction

The boom in triathlon (swimming, cycling, running competition) led to an increase in competition that accommodates multi-sport participants. The birth of multi-sport competition as a major participation sport led to the birth of multi-sport training.

a long-term exercise programme made up of different activities and sports

Triathlon involves swimming, cycling and running and is now an Olympic sport; biathlon involves swimming and running, and duathlon involves cycling and running. These competitions are now advertised in popular running, cycling and fitness magazines and include a number of distances to accommodate all levels from beginner to seasoned athlete. Further variety is provided by changing the cycling leg, traditionally a road time-trial section, to a mountain bike section, or changing the run from a road run to a cross-country run. In some events a kayak or sailing section is included as well as or instead of the swimming. Also increasing in popularity is adventure racing, involving outdoor activities such as fell running, walking, climbing, kayaking, skiing, mountain biking and horse riding: competitive multi-sport training for the outdoor enthusiast and survival specialist.

Preparing for these events requires that the participant train in each different sport involved. From a physiological perspective this ensures that all aspects of fitness are covered, whereas often one component of fitness is addressed and another ignored. So from these multi-sport events, was born multi-sport training, a long-term exercise programme made up of different activities and sports in order to provide variety and reduce the risk of injury whilst improving all-round fitness.

A multi-sport training programme may include competitive sports, outdoor activities such as those already mentioned and indoor fitness activities such as weight training and aerobics. The appeal of multi-sport training is in the variety of exercise in the programme, which serves to maintain long term interest and to tax different muscle groups in different ways. One day the participant may run, putting greater stress on the muscles and joints of the legs, and the next day may swim, reducing the impact on the joints and working the upper body more.

'Everyone has limits on the time they can devote to exercise, and multi-sport training simply gives you the best return on your investment. Balanced fitness with minimum injury risk and maximum fun.'

Top triathlete Paula Newby-Fraser

Who is it for?

Multi-sport training is for everyone. No matter what a person's age or level of fitness, anyone who wants balanced, all-round fitness and enjoys a variety of activities will benefit from and enjoy multi-sport training.

I run and weight train. Why do I need to multi-sport train as well?

If you run and weight train you are already multi-sport training. Running works your cardiovascular system and develops muscular endurance in the legs. Weight training works on muscular strength and endurance in your upper body, so your training programme may be more balanced than if you simply run or simply weight train. Most people who work out in clubs multi-sport train using CV machines such as treadmills, steppers, rowing machines, static bikes etc. to improve their aerobic fitness, and using resistance equipment to work on muscular strength.

Many people combine weights or resistance training indoors with walking, running or cycling outdoors to the same effect. Combining different activities utilises different parts of the body, different combinations of muscles, and even different combinations of muscle fibres within a muscle. This does not happen to the same extent in single-activity training; overall a more balanced fitness programme emerges.

Is multi-sport training OK for young athletes?

Most experts recommend that before puberty children participate in a variety of sports rather than specialising, even if a particular talent is discovered at an early age. Too early specialisation may result in 'burn out' or in overuse injury. Injury prevention is particularly important in growing children, who should be supervised by a trained coach or instructor with specialist knowledge of coaching children. Careful monitoring of training will help protect against the possibility of serious injuries occurring to bone growth centres. This makes multi-sport training particularly suitable for young athletes because full and rounded development is encouraged by participation in a number of different activities, each putting different stresses on the body.

Is multi-sport training useful for competitive sports people?

The more highly trained an athlete becomes the more difficult it is to improve performance. In relative beginners, or those less dedicated to training, improvements to any physiological area may improve performance in any one sport. For the athlete who is seriously dedicated to high-level competitive sport, then specificity of training becomes more of an issue. For these athletes multi-sport training is unlikely to improve performance in a single sport: the training must be focused on and specific to that sport to allow for the tiny improvements in performance that may make the difference between winning and losing.

What are the benefits of multi-sport training?

Multi-sport training and health

The well-researched and documented health benefits associated with exercise are only apparent in those who exercise regularly and long term. Statistics show that

'Multi-sport training is not the key to performing a specific sport at your best. Training in that sport is.

In a perfect world, with perfect bodies and no other stresses, we would not need to multi-sport train. So why do it? Because as mere mortals, our bodies get injured, our minds gets tired, and our schedules get hectic.

So, multi-sport train to maintain muscular balance and avoid injury. Multi-sport train to correct specific muscular weaknesses. Multi-sport train when time constraints keep you from doing your primary sport, but your body still needs work. Multi-sport train to work your body while resting your mind. In other words, use cross training as a means to an end, always remembering your primary performance goal, and the specific training it requires.'

Stephen Seiler, Associate Professor at the Institute of Health and Sport,
Agder College, Kristiansand, Norway.

most people who start an exercise programme drop out within the first three months.[1] Even in supervised exercise programmes the drop-out rate is around 50%.[2] Cross training can provide variety which may prevent the boredom often associated with continuing an exercise programme.

Injury prevention

Studies have shown that overuse injuries are associated with an increased volume of training, and that injuries in runners are related to increased weekly mileage and/or frequency of running or racing. Runners who do not participate in any other sport are more likely to become injured.[3] By changing the activity regularly and thus reducing the repetition of movement, multi-sport training allows for the greater levels of fitness brought about by increases in training volume without a concomitant increase in the risk of injury.

Some people stop exercising because as they increase their activity levels they pick

A study on runners evaluated increased risk of injury with respect to gender

* age
* obesity
* weekly mileage
* time per mile during training
* time and place of running
* stretching habits of the of participants.

It was concluded that only weekly mileage was positively associated with increased incidence of injury.[4] A study on aerobics class participants showed that injury risk was greater in those who participated in aerobic exercise only once per week and in those who did no other sport.[5]

up an injury. Because they have to stop doing their chosen activity, temporarily or permanently, they fail to get back into a regular exercise routine or simply give up exercising, believing that the injury has prevented it.

Single-activity participants often show imbalances of muscle strength, muscle mass, and flexibility. For instance the quadriceps muscles at the front of the thigh are often visibly larger on the dominant leg (i.e. the leg most commonly lunged on) in squash players. Likewise tennis players often have greater muscle mass in the playing arm than in the non-playing arm. Imbalances of muscular strength, muscle mass, and flexibility can lead to injury. As multi-sport training utilises different disciplines these imbalances are less likely to occur in multi-sport than in single-activity participants.

Many sportspeople who become injured simply give up exercise until their injury is healed. This time of complete rest, whilst accommodating the recovery from the injury sets back their training programme dramatically. A multi-sport training programme, because it uses different sports and therefore puts different stresses on the muscle and joint complexes maintains fitness whilst the injury is healing.

One personal training client of mine, unable to continue her sport of distance running whilst recovering from a stress fracture in her foot, maintained her cardiovascular fitness and aerobic capacity by cycling and swimming. Only two weeks after she started to run again she ran a personal best in a 10-kilometre race.

Maintenance of fitness through multi-sport training not only reduces the time spent reaching playing fitness again after injury, but may speed up the healing process by reducing muscle loss, strengthening the injured area and correcting any muscular imbalances. Whilst continuing to train, the stress on the injured area can gradually be increased as healing takes place and the new tissue becomes stronger or the joint becomes more stable.

Balanced fitness

When individuals successfully meet the challenge of exercise during the preparation for and participation in sport they do so as a result of an exquisitely orchestrated collection of physiological and metabolic events.

Professor Clyde Williams

Whether training for general fitness and health or for sports performance the words of Prof. Clyde Williams are true. The body is a fascinating machine, beautiful in its complexity. It is a machine not only in which physiological and metabolic events interact, but psychological aspects such as motivation and mental attitude play an important role in influencing outcomes, whether that be high-level performance or simply the motivation to move.

However, this 'exquisitely orchestrated collection of physiological and metabolic events' can 'get out of tune'. In order to play the perfect symphony our training must be geared to making the most of all aspects of fitness, so to multi-sport train effectively we must first understand at least a little about the orchestra and how its different sections play together. Physical fitness is the integration and balance of a variety of components affecting the cardiovascular and pulmonary systems (the

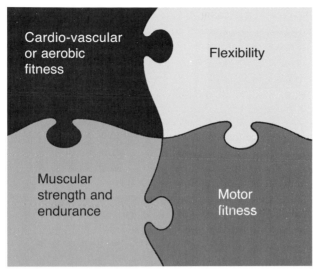

Figure 1.1 *Physical fitness*

heart and lungs), the skeleton and joints, the muscles, and the nervous system. To obtain all-round fitness, all aspects of fitness must be trained.

Why is training good for my heart and lungs?

Cardiovascular fitness refers to the condition of the heart and circulatory system. Training that is endurance based such as walking, running, swimming, rowing, canoeing, skating, skipping and dancing affect the heart increasing its size, strength and function such that there is an increase in **stroke volume** and **cardiac output**. That is, more blood is pumped out of the heart at every single beat. This has the effect of reducing the pulse rate both at rest and at various intensities of exercise, thus at any given intensity the heart beats more slowly in a trained than in an untrained individual and during exhaustive exercise the cardiac output is greater in the trained than in the untrained individual. This greater cardiac output is often attributed to the increase in size of the heart. In reality the increase in size is minimal and the increased cardiac output is largely the result of greater filling of the ventricles that results in a greater stroke volume.

Blood carries

- oxygen
- foodstuffs
- enzymes
- hormones
- waste products
- heat

- With the right type of training the improvements in the heart are accompanied by improvements to the general circulation – the blood transport system. There is an

Stroke volume is the amount of blood ejected from the left ventricle of the heart during contraction.

Cardiac output is the volume of blood per minute pumped by the heart and is the stroke volume times the heart rate.

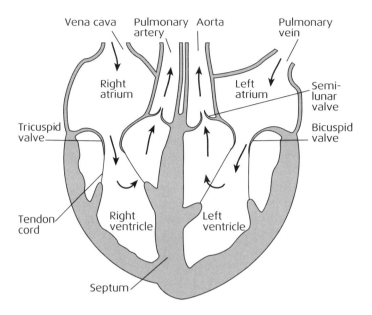

Figure 1.2. The heart

increase in the size and number of **capillaries** flowing through the regularly worked muscles. This allows the body to transport oxygen, nutrients, **hormones** and **enzymes** to the muscle and waste products away from the muscle more effectively.

> **Capillaries** are small blood vessels forming a network throughout the body.
> **Hormones** are chemical messengers produced by the body and transported in the blood to its target tissue.
> **Enzyme** is a complex protein formed in living cells and assisting chemical processes without being changed itself, i.e. organic catalysts.

- **Blood pressure** is the pressure that the blood exerts on the walls of the blood vessels. Thus an increase in the size and number of capillaries will decrease blood pressure both at rest and at work. Blood pressure at rest and during submaximal exercise decreases as a result of regular aerobic training.

> **Blood pressure** is written as two numbers, e.g. 140/90. The larger number is systolic blood pressure or the pressure during systole when the heart is contracting. The smaller number is diastolic blood pressure or the pressure during diastole when the heart is relaxing. Normal blood pressure is often quoted as 120/80, though a range from 110/60 to 140/90 is usually accepted as normal. If blood pressure is consistently above 160/90 you should consult your doctor.

- Oxygen is carried in the blood in association with **haemoglobin**. Haemoglobin, found in red blood cells, is a protein pigment containing iron. Every haemoglobin

> **Haemoglobin** is the iron-containing pigment of red blood cells that carries oxygen in the blood.
> **Myoglobin** is a pigment found in muscle that transports oxygen from the cell membrane to the mitochondria.

molecule can carry four oxygen molecules. When the oxygen reaches the muscle it is given up by the haemoglobin and diffuses across the cell membranes and into the muscle where it is carried on another protein pigment called **myoglobin**. Endurance training causes an increase in total blood volume and also in total haemoglobin levels in the blood. This improves the oxygen-carrying capacity of the blood. There is also an increase in the myoglobin content of the working muscle.

- The lungs are the site of gaseous exchange. In the lungs oxygen enters the bloodstream from the air, and carbon dioxide, a by-product of the aerobic energy system, leaves the blood and is released back into the air. Regular endurance training improves the function of the lungs, by increasing the power and endurance of the intercostal muscles and the diaphragm. Breathing occurs when the lungs are inflated and deflated like bellows. This is controlled by the muscle of the diaphragm, which spans the bottom of the ribcage, and the intercostal muscles between the ribs. Endurance training improves the function of these muscles and is associated with an increase in breathing volume. This higher maximum ventilation is a result of increases in both breathing frequency and **tidal volume**.

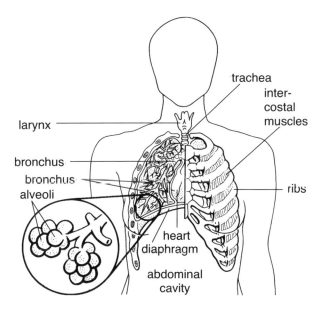

Figure 1.3 The lungs

Why is training good for my muscles?

Regular training of any kind will improve the function of muscles. Muscles rarely work in isolation. They may be causing movement around a joint or joints, they may be stabilising the body position or they may be checking movement at a joint in order to prevent injury. Whatever the job of the muscle in any particular movement or posture, both strength and endurance of that muscle or group of muscles may be involved. Maximum strength is the ability of a muscle or group of muscles to overcome a resistance once. Endurance is the ability of a muscle or group of muscles to overcome a resistance for an extended period of time, that is more than once.

> Increases both in strength and in endurance of the muscles may benefit **health** by accommodating safe lifting and maintaining the integrity of the joints during movement.
>
> Increases both in strength and in endurance of the muscles may benefit **sports performance** by increasing the total work capacity of the muscle either in terms of volume or intensity or both.

> **Tidal volume** is the amount of air that is moved in or out of the lungs in one breath.
>
> Improvements in the lungs also include greater capilliarization, that is an increase in the size and number of blood vessels in the lungs which increases the capacity for gaseous exchange.

Why is training good for my skeleton?

Osteoporosis is a medical condition often known as brittle bone disease because the bones become fragile and in severe cases may fracture spontaneously. Although this disease mainly affects women the number of men also affected is growing.

The skeleton is made up of living tissue. If the skeleton is not worked it will become weak in the same way that unused muscle becomes weak. Where the skeleton is subjected to forces it will become stronger. However, even in terms of skeletal strength, training is specific. Only those parts of the skeleton subjected to force will become stronger, thus a runner may have strong bones in the legs and hips but may not have strong bones in the forearms and wrists, and

> By the age of 60 one woman in four has fractures related to osteoporosis; this becomes one in two by the age of 70[6].

a tennis player may have greater strength in the bones in the playing arm than in the non-playing arm. Strong bones are vital to health. The widespread incidence of **osteoporosis** is believed to be at least in part due to long-term lack of exercise. Other factors include diet, age, gender and genetics.

Why is training good for my joints?

Wherever two or more bones meet there is a joint. Joints come in a variety of types but those most involved with movement are synovial joints: these allow for varying

Osteoporosis is a medical condition often known as brittle bone disease because the bones become fragile and in severe cases may fracture spontaneously. Although this disease mainly affects women, the number of men affected is growing.

degrees of freedom of movement, determined by the shape of the joint. For instance hinge joints such as the elbow allow for movement in one plane only, whereas ball and socket joints, such as in the hip, allow for movement in three planes. The ball and socket joint allows for a large range of movement in any one plane, whereas the joints in between each vertebrae of the spine allow for only small ranges of movement.

Stabilising the joints are ligaments made up of connective tissue, and crossing the joints are muscles that affect the movement or increase the stabilisation of the joint by holding it still or by counteracting a movement. Training may increase the strength of the stabilising muscles and also increase the strength of ligaments, thus maintaining the integrity of the joint during applications of force, such as when landing from a jump.

Why is training good for my nervous system?

The nervous system is the control centre for the body. Any movement involves contracting individual muscle fibres or groups of muscle fibres in the right sequence to cause that movement to happen. Simultaneously opposing muscle fibres must be allowed to relax in order that they do not block that movement from happening. This is known as reciprocal innervation. The nervous system controls the contraction and relaxation of muscle fibres and so is in charge of the combinations and

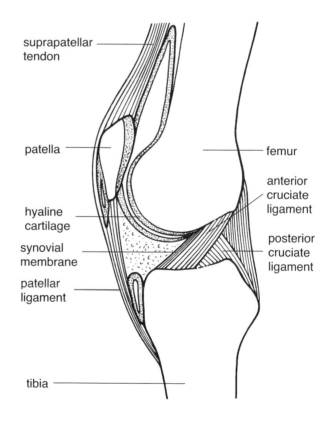

Figure 1.4 Synovial joints

- suprapatellar tendon
- patella
- hyaline cartilage
- synovial membrane
- patellar ligament
- tibia
- femur
- anterior cruciate ligament
- posterior cruciate ligament

sequences, both intramuscularly (within a muscle) and intermuscularly (between different muscles or groups of muscles). Learning the correct sequences of intra- and intermuscular contraction to carry out a movement is the acquisition of skill, so learning a physical skill involves training the nervous system. As the body tires so does the nervous system, and skill is reduced. Training the body for endurance has the effect of increasing the endurance of the nervous system as well as of muscles.

Freedom of movement

The joints and the muscles accommodate ease of movement. Flexibility is joint-specific, that is, it may be different for each individual joint or joint complex. It is possible to have a good range of movement in the shoulder joints and poor range of movement in the hips, for instance. Range of movement is affected by the shape of the joint, the connective tissues such as ligaments and joint capsules, the muscles crossing the joint, and the skin. As we age we tend to become less flexible. By continuing to be active and to train flexibility, we can, however, reduce the loss in flexibility and maintain ease of movement. Flexibility training should therefore be an integral part of every training programme.

How much training should I do?

The answer depends very much on what you wish to get out of your training. Do you simply want to be healthy or do you want to compete at a sport? If your main aim is to improve your health or remain healthy then you need do far less training than if you play sport. If you wish to take part in some type of activity such as hill walking, climbing, sailing or wind surfing, even if you consider that the activity is for fun rather than competitive, you will need to be fitter than is necessary just to maintain health.

Are there any recommended guidelines for fitness?

Table 1.1 Suggested Guidelines

Health	Fitness	Sport
Moderate intensity activity such as a brisk walk for 30–60 min on most days of the week	Aerobic activity 20 min three times per week at 50–90% VO_2max. Strength work twice a week using 1 or 2 sets of 8–10 reps of 8–10 exercises using the whole body	Training should be specific and allow to peak for specific events

The American College of Sports Medicine issues guidelines for fitness that are widely accepted throughout the world. They state that frequency of cardio-respiratory training should be 3–5 days per week at an intensity of 55/65–90 per cent of maximum heart rate, or 40/50–85 per cent of maximum oxygen uptake. (The lower intensity values, i.e. 55–64 per cent of HRmax and 40–49 per cent of VO_2max, are most applicable to individuals who are quite unfit.) Training should be for a duration of 20–60 min of continuous or intermittent aerobic activity (short bouts may be accumulated during the day but each bout should be a minimum of 10 min). Duration is dependent on the intensity of the activity: lower-intensity activity should be conducted over a longer period of time (30 min or more), and individuals training at higher levels of intensity should train at least 20 min or longer. The activity should use large muscle groups and should be maintained continuously. It should be rhythmical and aerobic in nature, for example walking-hiking, running-jogging, cycling, cross-country skiing, aerobic dance/group exercise, rope skipping, rowing, stair climbing, swimming, skating, and various endurance game activities or some combination thereof.

The ACSM states that resistance training should also be an integral part of an adult fitness programme and be of a sufficient intensity to enhance strength and muscular endurance and maintain fat-free mass (FFM). Resistance training should be progressive in nature, individualised, and provide a stimulus to all the major muscle groups. One set of 8–10 exercises, 8–12 repetitions, conditioning the major muscle groups, carried out 2–3 days per week is recommended. Most people should complete 8–12 repetitions of each exercise.

Flexibility exercises should be incorporated into the overall fitness programme sufficient to develop and maintain range of motion (ROM). Static and/or dynamic exercises stretching the major muscle groups should be performed a minimum of 2–3 days per week.[7]

Physical Activity and Health, A Report of the Surgeon General is widely used as a reference document and restates the ACSM guidelines.[8]

> All people over the age of 2 should accumulate at least 30 minutes of endurance-type activity of at least moderate intensity on most – preferably all – days of the week.
>
> Additional health and functional benefits of physical activity can be achieved by adding more time in moderate intensity activity, or by substituting more vigorous intensity activity.

The report of the Surgeon General goes on to say that:

> Strength development activities (resistance training) should be performed at least twice per week. At least 8–10 strength developing exercises that use the major muscle groups of the legs, trunk, arms and shoulders should be performed at each session, with one or two sets of 8–12 repetitions of each exercise.

Of course following the guidelines on minimum levels of fitness for health will not equip you for sports performance. To play sport we need to examine the demands of the sports and base fitness training on these demands.

Part II
How to get started

Common multi-sport training activities

Many people multi-sport train within a gym or health club environment using treadmills, rowers, steppers and stationary bikes together with resistance machines or free weights either during the same workout or during separate workouts. The cardiovascular machines provide training for the cardio-respiratory system, i.e. the heart and lungs, and endurance for the muscles, whereas the fixed resistance or free weights training complements this with increased strength and muscular endurance. By adding flexibility, good all-round physical fitness training is accommodated.

Some other common multi-sport training mixes choose from walking, swimming, running, rowing, paddling, cycling or aerobic dance to provide cardiovascular training and add strength work in the form of weight or circuit training. Some programmes aim to accommodate adherence to cardiovascular training better by mixing different cardiovascular sports, such as running and cycling or running and swimming, or commonly all three. As with all forms of training, multi-sport training becomes far more effective if it is planned.

Adding in flexibility

Some sports, notably martial arts, dancing and gymnastics, which are reliant on high degrees of flexibility for performance, incorporate a lot of flexibility work into their training; therefore, including these sports as a non-competitive element of a programme may be of benefit. Runners, for instance, may benefit greatly from participating in t'ai chi. Many bodybuilders benefit from dance training for both the flexibility work and for the grace and body awareness needed for posing routines. Regardless of the activity or sport, every programme should include flexibility training. Flexibility training ensures that we can move easily and that we are able to twist, turn and reach, thus enhancing sports performance, improving posture and protecting against injury in everyday life as well as when taking part in sports.

Most experts agree that during warm-up for any exercise or sport it is advisable to put the joints through a full range of movement. It is also agreed that immediately following exercise or sport, as part of the cool-down, one should stretch the muscles that have been worked. However, stretching exercises can also be done at other times, sitting in front of the fire in the evening, for instance, or in small bursts at any time during the day.

How do I know what to choose in my training programme?

By and large, choose activities or sports that you enjoy; that way you will be more likely to keep training. As your tastes change, change your training activities.

Some activities are complementary to each other. For instance weight training, if done correctly, may enhance rowing performance. Cycling may improve or maintain running performance on fewer running miles. Kayaking may add a wet-weather sport to the repertoire for someone who participates in a dry-weather sport such as rock climbing.

If your sports are all heavily reliant on the legs – cycling and running for instance – you may look at a sport that involves more upper body work, such as weight training, swimming or kayaking. If your sports are very endurance-based, such as long distance running or hill walking, you may wish to add a sport that is more strength/endurance- and skill-based such as rock climbing or windsurfing. If your sport is highly intensive you may find a lower-intensity sport that is complementary, for instance an ice hockey player may take up walking.

Much depends on what exactly you want to get out of your multi-sport training programme.

Multi-sport training and sport

Decathlon, heptathlon, and pentathlon have long provided multi-discipline competition, while traditionally, depending on the season, many cyclists and runners at club level and above have competed in road, track and cross country events, each of which provide a slightly different challenge. It was, however, the sudden upsurge of interest in swimming, cycling and running competition, the birth of triathlon that heralded a new era in which multidiscipline sports increased in popularity.

What is triathlon ?

Triathlon is a three-discipline sports competition, normally a combination of swimming, cycling and running. Two competitive distances have become popular: Olympic distance, entailing a 1000-metre swim, a 40-kilometre cycle section and a 10-kilometre run, and iron man, with a 2-mile swim, a 72-mile bike ride and a full marathon distance 26.2-mile run. Other distances are put together to provide sprint triathlons, half iron man and ultra iron man events. Biathlons involving swimming and running and duathlon with a run - bike - run format are also popular.

The UK Ultra-Fit Challenge

- indoor cycle 1 kilometre
- indoor row 500 metres
- lat pulldown 40 reps (resistance machine)
- step-ups 100 reps
- press-ups 60 reps
- sit-ups 60 reps
- overhead press 40 reps (resistance machine)
- treadmill run 800 metres 10% incline
- bench press 40 reps (free weight)

Other multi-sport competitions

Triathlons involving other sports are also becoming popular, for instance indoor rowing on a rowing **ergometer** such as the Concept II is often combined with a track cycle section and a track run.

Indoor Multi-sport Training Challenge competitions such as the 'Ultrafit' competition have increased in popularity with gym and health-club members. These involve disciplines drawn from a combination of cardiovascular machines, callisthenics and resistance equipment.

> **Ergometer** – a piece of equipment that is calibrated and produces measurable units of work such that a person's work output can be measured

For outdoor athletes, kayaking, mountain biking and fell running have become a popular competitive combination. Often marketed as a form of triathlon, it has paved the way for adventure sports that incorporate a combination of events from such disciplines as running, kayaking, sailing, mountain biking, climbing, riding, cross-country skiing and mountaineering. Challenges such as the Raid Gauloises, the Eco Challenge and the Southern Traverse attract elite athletes with major sponsorship.

Adventure races are most usually team events, often the whole team completing the whole course. Sometimes they run as a relay and occasionally as single-competitor events.

The Count Down has Begun
Saturday, November 8th, 1997 – 9 a.m. NZT

Geoff & Pascal have begun what must be one of the most hectic weeks anyone could ask for. Last minute preparations, the arrival of international guests and media, a million photocopies, volunteers to organise, and on and on it goes. So too for the competitors who will be anxiously checking equipment, organising their support crews and hoping that these months of hard training are going to be sufficient for what lies ahead. The course is still a highly guarded secret so if you want to find out first I suggest you stay online for the first official release.

This afternoon teams were given a competency test on the ropes rigged up at a local resort in preparation for the new abseiling section of the course. Following this the local college was transformed into briefing HQ where the starting point was revealed for the first time. Competitors listened nervously as the long-range weather forecast was read out warning of very cold temperatures, snow and high winds affecting most areas of the course.

Extract from report on the Southern Traverse 1997[1]

Do different modes of training combine to give as effective a training stimulus as single activities?

The question that many sports people ask is whether cross training will improve their performance. Scientific research has also asked this question: can one compare the effectiveness of different types of training activities? One study investigated the changes in aerobic capacity in moderately active college-aged students and discovered similar improvements in **VO₂max** achieved with running and with in-line skating programmes, provided that the training programmes were equivalent in volume and intensity.[2]

In another study moderately fit runners trained four days per week in either run-only sessions or alternating run and cycle training at 85–90 per cent maximum heart rate. Both groups significantly improved VO_2max and run performance over 5000 metres with no difference between groups.[3]

VO_2max is the highest amount of oxygen that the body can consume for the aerobic production of ATP. That is the amount of oxygen that the body can take in and utilise in the working muscles for the production of energy.

It would seem from the research available that some transfer of training effects on maximum oxygen uptake (VO_2max) exists from one training mode to another. This however seems to be more noticeable when running is performed as a multi-sport training mode, while swim training may result in minimum transfer of training effects on VO_2max.[4] This may be due to swim training being non-weight-bearing and an activity that utilises the smaller muscles of the upper body extensively, whereas run training is weight-bearing and utilises the large muscles of the legs. If this is the case then one would suppose that activities such as in-line skating would have similar transfer of training effects to that of running so long as both training modes activated similar neural firing patterns and force velocity characteristics. For this reason cross-country skiers often use uphill walking as a training activity in preference to running. For activities that rely on high levels of maximum oxygen uptake, that is, endurance-based events, it would therefore seem that appropriate types of multi-sport training, that is, training that utilises the same muscle groups in the same way, may have a significant effect on VO_2max; however, this training effect never exceeds those induced by sport-specific training, that is, single-discipline training.

Interval training consists of intermittent exercise with regular rest periods between the work periods. The ratio of **work** to **rest** is manipulated according to the desired training effect.

Multi-sport training may also have some crossover effect between physiological adaptations. For instance, one study showed that during nine weeks of an aerobic **interval training** programme of 3 min **work** intervals at 90 per cent VO_2max and 3 min **rest** intervals at 25-40 per cent VO_2max, anaerobic power improved and performance in repeated high-intensity short-duration work increased.[5] That is, the high-intensity aerobic training had a small but nevertheless significant training effect on anaerobic ability, the ability to perform very high intensity short-duration work such as sprinting.

> **High-intensity aerobic training** has a small but nevertheless significant training effect on the ability to perform very high intensity short-duration work such as sprinting.

Improvements in physiology do not always equate to improved performance. Each sport entails a unique combination of demands such as skill, high VO_2max, high **anaerobic threshold** level, high peak power, sustainable power output, psychological ability, etc. It is the combination of these factors that enables sports people to perform at their best. If VO_2max is not the competitor's limiting factor then although training may help the individual to improve his or her VO_2max it may not result in improved performance.

> **anaerobic threshold** – also called 'onset of blood lactate accumulation' (OBLA) or lactate threshold – is the workload at which lactate production is greater than lactate removal and so lactate builds up to a level where muscular contraction is interfered with.

For instance, swimmers may include running in their programme and as a result may improve their VO_2max. However, if it is their muscular endurance in the arms and shoulders that is limiting their performance, they will not improve as a result of run training. A cyclist may multi-sport train by running or skating to improve VO_2max, but if power output on the hills is the limit to performance, again performance will not improve subsequent to running training. The more highly trained an athlete becomes the more difficult it is to improve performance. In relative beginners to sports, or those less dedicated to training, improvements to any physiological area may improve performance in any one sport.

> For the athlete who is more dedicated to regular serious training multi-sport training is unlikely to improve performance in a single sport. Rather the training must be focused on and specific to that sport to allow for the tiny improvements in performance that may make the difference between winning and losing.

So why should a single-sport athlete multi-sport train?

For the single-sport athlete multi-sport training my provide some psychological relief and provide a way of maintaining fitness while reducing the mechanical stresses on the body that are normally associated with high-volume single-sport training.

For the injured athlete multi-sport training may help maintain fitness while resting the injury and allowing for recovery.

For some athletes multi-sport training provides for times when they are unable to participate in their sport. For instance, ice skaters and ice hockey players are restricted to specific rink times. They need to train off the ice as well if they are to get the best from their training programme.

Do strength and endurance training successfully combine?

Many endurance athletes in the past have shied away from strength training, believing that excess muscle development will increase their body weight and negatively impact their endurance performance. It is well recognised, however, that increases in strength often have a positive effect on endurance performance and are not necessarily accompanied by large increases in muscle bulk. This was demonstrated in one scientific study in which a combination of heavy resistance training and distance running training improved running economy in serious female recreational runners when compared to a similar group who performed running training alone.[6] Likewise when studying the strength gains made in females who also underwent endurance training it was found there was no impairment of strength development although the same muscles were used in the endurance training activity.[7]

- For the general population, cross training may be highly beneficial in terms of overall fitness.

- The principles of specificity of training tend to have greater significance, especially for highly trained athletes.

- Similarly, cross-training may be an appropriate supplement during rehabilitation periods from physical injury and during periods of overtraining or psychological fatigue.

It does, however, seem evident from the studies done to date that, as with many aspects of training, there is no simple answer to the questions raised regarding the mixing of strength and endurance activities. There is other evidence that high-volume, high-intensity strength training may impair development of high levels of aerobic endurance and that **muscular hypertrophy** and development of high levels of absolute strength may be inhibited by high-volume, high-intensity aerobic training.

Muscular hypertrophy is the increase of muscle mass that occurs when the muscle filaments undergo change following resistance work, often heavy weight training.

The body is complex and so training it will also be complex. Whereas for most people multi-sport training has a positive effect on fitness, elite athletes wishing to be competitive at the top end of a single-discipline sport must be sure of the reasons why they are multi-sport training before they embark on a programme. At the top level for single-sport athletes multi-sport training will not in itself improve performance, rather training should be specific if it is to increase performance gains. However, if multi-sport training keeps the athlete in the sport, keeps him or her training, for instance by minimising muscle imbalances or injury risk, it may indirectly result in improved performance.

Summary of the advantages and disadvantages of training

Advantages

- Multi-sport training is an appropriate form of training for all-round fitness for most individuals.

- Multi-sport participants need to multi-sport train in the disciplines that are found in their sport.

- Single-sport competitors may benefit from multi-sport training in the form of injury prevention and rehabilitation. However, specific training will yield higher levels of sports performance for elite athletes.

- Strength and endurance training are mutually compatible and mutually beneficial for most people.

Disadvantages

- High-volume, high-intensity strength training may inhibit development of high levels of aerobic endurance.

- High-volume, high-intensity aerobic training may inhibit development of high levels of absolute strength or muscular hypertrophy.

Kitting yourself out for training

Each individual sport has specialist equipment, clothing and shoes. There is no doubt that having the right equipment for the job makes participating in the sport a lot more comfortable and often more enjoyable, and this would seem to make multi-sport training very expensive. Clearly, if you wish to cycle and kayak you need a bike and a kayak, both of which are expensive items.

There are, however, ways that you can reduce the overall cost of multi-sport training. For instance, outdoor clothing, used by fell runners and walkers and climbers is just as suitable to run in and, with the addition of padded shorts, to cycle in. If you normally use flat pedals rather than pedals requiring cleats you can cycle in running shoes or even hiking boots.

It is surprising how well our bodies can adapt to not having exactly the recommended clothing for a sport. Watch any triathlon and you will see many of the competitors exit from the water, put their cycling shoes on without socks, and head off to cycle anything up to 112 miles in their swimming costume and then, changing their cycling shoes for running shoes, still without socks, will run anything up to 26.2 miles in their swimming costume.

Look at the demands of the sport. Do you need to keep warm in cold or wet weather? Do you need clothing that will wick away sweat and dry extremely quickly? Do you need to keep dry and protected from the wind? Do you need to be able to add or reduce ventilation? Clothing is specifically designed by manufacturers to meet the needs of sportspeople – and then is heavily influenced by the fashion for each sport at that time. Often clothing is perfectly suitable for more than one sport, though you may not feel the part running in your cycling jersey. Gradually, as you find which sports and what type of equipment suits you, you will probably collect specialist clothing for each sport that you partake in.

Having chosen your activities, or at least found two activities that you wish to include in your training, the next thing to do is to start.

Beginners to exercise

If you are a complete beginner, or are returning to training after a long break, training is an excellent method of getting fit. Choose two or three sports in which you wish to take part and start as a complete beginner in all of them. However, you must be careful not to overload. You are less at risk of injury than if you start a training programme with just one sport, because you will be stressing different parts of the body at different times.

Aim to exercise three or four times per week and to alternate disciplines. Exercise at an intensity that is reasonably comfortable but provides more stress to the body than is normal for you.

Table 3.1 *12-week programme for walk and aerobics class*

Week 1	Week 2	Week 3	Week 4	Week 5	Week 6
Walk × 2	Walk × 2	Walk × 2	Walk × 3	Walk × 3	Walk × 3
Weights × 1	Weights × 1	Weights × 1	Weights × 1	Weights × 1	Weights × 1
Week 7	**Week 8**	**Week 9**	**Week 10**	**Week 11**	**Week 12**
Walk × 3	Walk × 3	Walk × 3	Walk × 3	Walk × 3	Walk × 3
Weights × 2	Weights × 2	Weights × 2	Weights × 2	Weights × 2	Weights × 2

Start by walking at about 75 per cent of maximum effort for 10 to 15 min and gradually increase until you are walking as fast as you can for 15 to 20 min. After the first six weeks for your third walk work at about 50 per cent of maximum effort but walk for about 45 min to an hour. As you progress, on this walk increase the distance or time that you are walking for, rather than the speed.

For each exercise use a weight for which you just complete 15 repetitions. Complete 15 repetitions at this weight for each session. As completing the set becomes easy, add a little weight on to that particular exercise.

Ab curls can be done on an ab machine or on the floor. A rest of 1–2 minutes should be taken between each set.

In week 1, use the weight that you were using for 15 repetitions and complete three sets of 10 repetitions with a rest in between each set. Gradually over the six weeks you may find that you can increase the weight on particular exercises. Increase to where you can just manage to perform all ten repetitions in the third set.

Table 3.2 Weights session, first 6 weeks

Exercise	Reps
Leg press/squats	15
Bench/chest press	15
Leg extensions	15
Lat pulldowns	15
Leg curls	15
Shoulder press	15
Leg abductions	15
Seated row	15
Leg adductions	15
Ab curls	15

Table 3.3 Weights programme for second six weeks

Exercise	Sets	Reps
Leg press/squats	3	10
Bench/chest press	3	10
Leg extensions	3	10
Lat pulldowns	3	10
Leg curls	3	10
Shoulder press	3	10
Leg abductions	3	10
Seated row	3	10
Leg adductions	3	10
Ab curls	3	15

For the more experienced

First you should look at why you want to multi-sport train. If you are generally a single-sport athlete and you want to keep your main sport but balance your fitness training, then this sport will remain as the basis of your training with the other activities complementing the programme.

If you wish to use multi-sport training to ensure all-round fitness and to add variety to your programme then you need only look at the overall balance of your programme.

As a single-sport athlete, choose one or two sports that complement your original one. If you are competitive, try to start your multi-sport training in your rest season, or just after a major competition, and ease into it. The main focus should be to enjoy yourself.

You will probably need to cut down on your training volume for your main sport at least temporarily to give yourself the time to add in the new sport(s) and to ensure you do not overstress your body. Add in one sport at a time. As you will be using different muscles, or the same muscles in a different way, or different muscle fibres and different firing patterns within a muscle, expect that the new sport will be tiring at first.

If you are not a single-sport athlete but are wanting to multi-sport train for all-round fitness then choose which sports you want to include and a level that is reasonably comfortable to start with, and work from there. You may find that you want to take part in organised multidiscipline activities or competitions or that you like to do different activities at different times of the year. Enjoy experimenting with your sport to find what works best for you.

If you are already training regularly then just start on a multi-sport training programme by doing something different, and as you read later in this book about programming you can organise your training more scientifically. There are sample programmes for both single-sport athletes using multi-sport training to balance their sport and for multi-sport athletes in chapter 20.

④ Warm-up and cool-down

Warming up

If you put a mixture of chemicals into a test tube and wait, normally a reaction will happen more quickly and easily if the test tube is warm. The body is similar. Generally it works better after a warm-up.

Increasing efficiency and reducing the risk of injury

During exercise the muscles demand an increase in the blood supply. This is partly met by greater cardiac output due to an increase in heart rate and partly by redirection of blood to the working muscles.

Like the test-tube experiment, the chemical reactions in the body that take place during exercise are speeded up if the body is warm. Muscle and connective tissue making up tendons and ligaments are pliable. These structures become more pliable when warm. A warm-up also facilitates the response of nervous tissue, meaning that activating fibres transmit impulses more quickly and feedback is more efficient.

These acute changes during warm-up for exercise increase the body's efficiency and reduce the chance of injury from inaccurate movement patterns, from tearing or straining cold muscles or from spraining joint structures.

Reducing build-up of lactic acid

At the start of exercise the sudden increases in demand for energy from the working muscles is met largely by the short term anaerobic supplies which are quick to respond. As exercise continues the contribution from the aerobic system gradually increases, characterised by an increase in both respiration rate and heart rate.

> If the energy demand at the onset of exercise is high, then large amounts of lactic acid build up in the cell and the anaerobic threshold is soon reached. Steady state may still occur, but with a higher residual level of lactic acid present. The residual level of lactic acid in the muscles may be close to threshold level. In this case even a slight rise in intensity of exercise, as may happen when running up a slight gradient, is likely to increase muscle lactate beyond threshold level, forcing the athlete to slow down.

At the onset of exercise, because the sudden increase in energy supply is largely dependent on the anaerobic systems, there is an increase in lactic acid production within the cells. Gradually the amount of energy supplied by the aerobic system increases to a point where it is able to meet the energy demand and the accumulated lactic acid is turned back into pyruvate and utilised as fuel. Steady state is reached.

A gradual and progressive warm-up may prevent this by allowing muscle lactate to clear so that a lower residual level is set when steady state is reached. After steady state is achieved, this will allow for small rises in intensity without crossing the anaerobic threshold.

Optimising energy supply from Fatty Acids

Lactic acid inhibits the utilisation of fat as fuel, forcing the muscle to use vital glycogen stores. Thus high residual levels of muscle lactate effectively drain the muscle glycogen stores, decreasing the ability to sustain long-duration exercise. Gradual progressive warm-up therefore allows for optimum usage of fat as fuel and optimum glycogen sparing.

What is the best way to warm up

Warm-up is really preparation for exercise. Warming-up should involve a gradual increase in the intensity of exercise, utilising the muscles that will be used during the sport and a gradual increase in the range of movement around the joints used in the sport. Clearly in some sports, such as cycling or resistance training on machines, the movement patterns are very regular and in other sports, such as fell running or training with free weights, they are far less so. Some sports, for instance gymnastics, require extreme ranges of movement. During the warm-up range of movement should gradually increase to simulate that likely to be used during the activity.

Once the muscles are warm a short period of stretching facilitates joint range and muscle lengthening. The intensity of exercise should then be gradually increased again until steady state is reached.

Cool-down

Cool-down might better be termed 'reparation'. The cool-down period exists gradually to disperse lactic acid from the muscles and to return contracted muscles to their resting state. If lactic acid has built up in the muscle cells it will be more quickly dispersed if exercise is continued at a reduced rate, thus allowing aerobic metabolism to use up some of the lactic acid and the blood pumping through the muscles to disperse the remainder more quickly.

Post-exercise stretching (cool-down stretch)

Some activities, such as gymnastics or some dance or martial arts training, may in themselves utilise a full range of movement; however, other activities use restricted ranges of movement. If the joints are never moved through their full ranges then reduced flexibility will ensue. Therefore stretching sessions are advisable as part of any training programme. As muscle is more pliable when warm, this is the time that it should be stretched, therefore it is customary to stretch after activity, while the muscles are warm and while one is still in training clothes that do not restrict range of movement.

This post-exercise stretch, sometimes termed 'cool-down stretch', in no way precludes the addition of specific stretching sessions to a programme, it simply ensures that after restricted range of movement activities the muscle is returned to its resting length and offers a convenient time to perform exercises aimed purely at increasing flexibility and range of movement.

When is a cool-down not a cool-down?

One should be warm to stretch. Thus after stop-and-go activities such as weight training it may be more appropriate to stretch the relevant parts of the body straight after each exercise, or to use a cardiovascular activity to warm up again in order that the muscles are warm enough to stretch after the training session.

By the same principle, when one is standing next to one's car in the freezing cold after a race, stretching should be kept to a minimum if done at all. In this instance one should at least put warm clothing on before stretching and should probably go home, have a warm bath and then stretch.

Post-exercise stiffness

There is much discussion on post-exercise stiffness. The fatigue that occurs directly at the end of strenuous exercise is most probably due to low glycogen stores, fatigued nerve pathways and a build-up of lactic acid. The lactic acid will disperse fairly quickly once exercise ceases, though restoring glycogen stores may take one or two days, depending on nutrition. The soreness that occurs in muscles during one or two days after an exercise session is delayed onset muscle soreness (DOMS), which is most probably due to a number of factors including micro-trauma in the muscle cells and leakage of enzymes, which then irritate the nerve endings. Depending on severity this trauma may take a few days to heal and the soreness may take a similar time to be relieved. Severe DOMS is a sign that the training session was too much for the training status of the athlete.

Multi-sport training and DOMS

DOMS is a symptom of muscle damage and injured muscles need to rest and heal. Multi sport training accommodates recovery without loss of fitness by offering alternative training that stresses different muscle fibres.

⑤ Running

As long as you are healthy you can start to run, but it is important to start gently and build up gradually. Contraindications to running as a training method include joint, back or muscular problems, recent surgery, pregnancy or having recently given birth. In these instances you should consult your doctor before you start.

What equipment do I need?

All you need to start is a pair of running shoes and comfortable clothing.

Clothing should not be heavy or impede movement, and should keep you warm in cold weather and cool in hot weather. Cotton T-shirts stay wet and so can become uncomfortable. Specialist running shops can provide you with clothing designed to wick away sweat.

Cold weather equipment

On cold days wear lots of thin layers rather than one thick layer. That way air is trapped in between the layers and acts as insulation; if you have too many layers you can strip off the top one and tie it round your waist or carry it in a bumbag. Start with a thin layer of thermal fabric next to the skin, followed by a warm synthetic such as a sweatshirt or fleece. On windy days in particular a windproof breathable outer layer is important. Each layer should allow perspiration to escape, so should be non-absorbent and quick to dry . There are many lightweight 'thermal' garments on the market designed for active lifestyles. While not essential they will help to ensure your comfort.

Gloves and a hat are advisable if the weather is very cold, as much heat is lost through the hands and head. If it is cold and raining you will chill very quickly unless you protect yourself from the wind, so a windproof outer layer is advisable. Again there are many varieties on the market. Try to avoid plastic garments, as these do not allow perspiration to escape. A waterproof, if required, should be made of a breathable fabric.

Warm weather equipment

On warm days choosing clothing is easy – simply wear whatever you are comfortable and cool in. Loose clothing allows air to circulate around the body and thus improves the body's ability to stay cool.

In strong sun a hat or visor may be advisable. A smear of petroleum jelly (such as Vaseline) across the forehead just above the eyebrows will prevent sweat from running into the eyes. Petroleum jelly is also useful to lubricate the top of the legs, under the arms or around the nipples to prevent chafing.

Footwear

Socks should be seam-free and should fit well. It may help to powder the feet lightly before running to guard against chafing or blisters.

Shoes are a matter of personal choice. Although most sports shops carry a small range of running shoes it worth going to a specialist running shop rather than buying from a regular sports shop unless you know what you are looking for. In a specialist shop the range of footwear will be larger and there should be someone who can advise you. You will find lists of such shops in running magazines stocked by newsagents. Try on a number of makes and models of shoe for comparison, and wear the socks that you intend to run in. The shoes must be comfortable in the shop, or they won't be comfortable to run in. You can't break running shoes in.

The shoe sole consists of a hardwearing outer sole, a midsole that absorbs shock, and a comfortable insole next to your feet.

Put on both shoes and lace them up. The heel counter should cradle the heel firmly so that the shoe does not slip, and the toebox should be roomy enough to allow the toes to swell a little without cramping them. Jump around in them. If the shop will let you, go for a test run.

There is much discussion about running shoes and the amount and type of impact absorption. Good running shoes are extremely comfortable: a friend of mine, when trying on a new pair of running shoes, said, 'It is like wearing cushions on your feet'.

'Wearers of expensive running shoes that are promoted as having additional features that protect (e.g., more cushioning, "pronation correction") are injured significantly more frequently than runners employing inexpensive shoes . . .

When habitually barefoot humans walk (and probably when they run), they have greater knee flexion, which has been shown to reduce shock . . .

..Although this may run counter to notions prevalent in economically advanced countries recounting dangers of barefoot activity and necessity of footwear even when barefoot activity is feasible, supporting data are lacking, and many have concluded that footwear design is guided by fashion rather than health considerations...

People who perform activities involving high impact while wearing footwear currently promoted as offering protection in this environment are at high risk of injury.'

Steven E. Robbins and Gerard J. Gouw,
'Athletic footwear: unsafe due to perceptual illusions',
Medicine and Science in Sport and Exercise, 23/2 (1991), 217–224[6].

Although this high comfort level is often used as a selling-point for sports shoes it is not necessarily a good thing. Research has shown that when the real impact load is greater than the perceived impact load, as occurs when shoes are well cushioned, the body fails to respond to the loading, thus injury is more likely to occur.

The type of running you intend to partake in will also play a significant role in choosing shoes. For instance, if practically all your running will be off-road, then fell running shoes may be far more suitable for you than road running shoes. If you train only on a track then racing flats may well be most suitable.

Whenever buying running shoes, be guided by what feels right on your feet.

Your first run

Running can be a sociable event, or a personal one. It can be easy or hard, competitive or friendly. You can run any time of the day, anywhere you happen to be, but the only way to start is to get your shoes on and get out there. Only you can make it happen!

Running is a very natural activity. Most people who try to start running and fail, do so because they set out too fast, they get out of breath, their muscles feel heavy or achy and refuse to work properly and they just stop and assume that they 'can't run'. The mistake they have made is to go too fast too soon.

Even if you regularly swim or cycle or attend aerobics class you may still find running hard work when you first try it. Setting out too fast employs the anaerobic energy systems and results in a build-up of lactic acid causing a feeling of heaviness in the legs, shortness of breath and a need to slow down. As with any other type of exercise a warm-up period is essential. Lack of preparation sets you up to fail. A warm-up, starting at low levels of intensity and gradually increasing, stimulates the body to speed up the heart rate, so pumping extra blood around the body.

Set off walking briskly and swinging your arms vigorously. Break into a slow jog, add a little easy skipping if you like, alternated with easy sidesteps (remembering to change the leading leg). Circle your shoulders, swing your arms, stop and mobilise your back by circling your hips. Gradually, as you warm up, increase your range of motion. If once you are running regularly you intend to add any speed work, on those sessions you will need to increase the range of motion until you are really striding out, although not yet at full speed.

Your level of fitness will determine your starting level. Listen to your body. Run at a pace at which you can hold a conversation. If you are getting too breathless to talk, slow down or walk until you have recovered, then set off again. Aim to run/walk for 10 minutes in total. That could be 5 minutes out and 5 minutes back or a circular route lasting 10 minutes. Run/walk every other day or every third day, gradually reducing the walking time and increasing the running time until you can run for the full ten minutes.

Now start to increase the running time by a minute or two every third session, until you can manage thirty minutes running. Even if you are feeling good, don't be tempted to increase your running time by more than about 10 per cent a week. Overuse injuries tend to sneak up on one unawares, and have a nasty habit of outstaying their welcome.

As you run you should put your heel down first and roll through to your toe. Try to keep your shoulders relaxed. Remember, although your breathing will be heavier than normal you should not be so out of breath that you can't talk.

You should run with fairly upright posture, leaning forwards only slightly.

At the end of each session you should 'warm down'. That means slowing down gradually and finishing with a slow jog or brisk walk until your heart rate and breathing return to more normal levels. Now, while you are still warm, is an ideal time to stretch well, paying special attention to the calves, hamstrings, quadriceps, hip flexors, and abductors. If it is cold weather try to get indoors to stretch.

Consistency and progression

Having been out for your first run you need to continue to run consistently and to progress in order to gain the benefits. Aim to run two or three times per week, making sure that you have a rest day between each running day. When you start to run just getting moving on a regular basis will improve your fitness levels. Eventually, however, there will come a time when you plateau. At that point further improvements will only come with smarter training following some well-founded training principles.

Many people run the same route at the same pace, or even different routes but at the same pace every time they run. Understandably they get bored with running, and because in reality we need to run at different intensities in order to train all aspects of our physiology, they reach a point where although they are maintaining healthy fitness levels they are not improving further.

The basis of any training programme is to manipulate frequency, intensity, time and type such that you make the best possible gains with the least risk of injury: 'Maximise the benefits, minimise the risks.' Frequency, intensity, time and type of training interact in such a way that it is impossible to lay down hard and fast rules around each area. Each individual has a genetic limit on the amount and intensity of training that they can handle before the body begins to break down, and superimposed upon this genetic limit is their present state of health and physical fitness, their current stress levels and their nutritional status.

The American College of Sports Medicine (ACSM) recommends training a minimum of three times a week aerobically and twice a week for strength in order to improve or maintain fitness. Further, they suggest that aerobic training should be at a minimum intensity equivalent to 60 per cent of maximum heart rate. Whereas these guidelines are very general, and as such are adequate for general fitness, they are not specific to any one individual or to that individual's goals. Nevertheless they provide a good starting-point for anyone on a maintenance programme or who simply wants to keep fit and be able to compete for fun and be able to finish an event.

Frequency

How frequently you should run depends on your goals, experience (that is how long you have been running for), health, age, and history of injury, as well, of course, as

If running is your first sport, decreasing your run training does not have to impact your central fitness. Although your run-specific fitness may need fine tuning once the injury is healed you will be able to keep your fitness levels high by multi-sport training using such sports as rowing or cycling while resting from running. I once broke my foot while training for a marathon. I missed the marathon but kept my fitness levels up by cycling and swimming. Once my foot had healed and I was able to run again, it took me only a couple of weeks to reach my previous performance levels over a half marathon distance.

how much time you have available.

If you have a history of injury you may need to alter your training. This may involve decreasing your running volume or changing the type of running that you do. For instance, you may need to run more on grass than on roads and other hard surfaces. Subsequently you might add in specific strength and flexibility work, extra skill work, body awareness or proprioreceptive training in order to strengthen the injured area and prepare for the rigours of training and competition with minimal risk of re-injury. Older athletes may be more prone to injury and may need to vary their training more. Younger athletes with immature bone and soft tissue development will be injury-prone if exposed to high training volumes in one single sport. They may be able to train often but for shorter periods of time only.

Proprioreceptive is the sensory information produced by sensory nerve cells which detect position of the body and its parts, extent and force of movement, muscular tension and physical pressure.

Intensity and duration

'Intensity' of exercise is most often measured by heart rate or by 'rate of perceived exertion' in the case of aerobic activity, though it may be measured by percentage of MVO_2 or by lactate levels. The intensity of the training interacts with the time or duration to stimulate different physiological improvements.

Even if the sole aim of running is to improve general fitness as part of a multi-sport training programme, greater benefit ensues from varying the intensity of the training. Sometimes one should train at low intensity for a long duration, sometimes at high intensity for a short duration.

Training intensity should be varied on different training sessions in order to get the most out of a training programme. The focus of the training intensity also depends on the physiological demands of the sport, the aim of the training sessions, the training, nutritional, health status of the athlete, the age of the athlete, the time available to train, and the length of the competitive year.

Mountain marathons that take two days to complete demand high levels of endurance at a relatively moderate intensity and therefore much of the training would be at low to moderate intensity but of long duration. Running 1500 metres also demands endurance, but for a shorter period of time and at very high intensity. Thus less of the training would be low intensity, long duration, and more sprint work would be needed to train for this event.

Your first fun run or race

You may start running as part of your multi-sport training programme and decide that you want to enter a fun run or race. Go and watch any 'fun run' and you will soon realise that this is serious stuff. Those at the front are out there trying to win, and many further back are just as seriously racing against the course, trying to beat last year's time or to set a new personal best. Don't they know this isn't a Commonwealth Games final? What is it all about?

Well, mostly it's about setting and achieving goals. For all but the most gifted of us, representing our country in the next Commonwealth Games is not even a dream away. On the other hand, finishing the local fun run is a distinct possibility. Hence at most races, even those with top-class performers, if there is open entry (that is, where anyone can enter, it is not by invitation only) there are as many, if not more, people simply finishing the race as there are running competitively.

How to choose a race

If you do not run at all and do NO exercise at the moment then deciding to run a marathon in a couple of months time is inadvisable. It may be a possibility, depending on how long it is since you exercised regularly, your genetics and your luck, but you will certainly give yourself a better chance of success if you choose a more modest achievement for your first race.

If you do no running at all right now, then to run 5 kilometres (3.1 miles) or 10 kilometres (6.2 miles) is a suitable goal. If, on the other hand, although you do not yet run you are an extremely fit cyclist, for instance, you may well be able to run a marathon within a couple of months. Assess your fitness levels in terms of how much training you now do and how long it is since you trained regularly. If you have not trained at all for a number of years give yourself longer to achieve the goal.

If you already run regularly you may want to decide on a race distance dependent on how much time you have to train and what distance you like to run. Inevitably to run a marathon or a half marathon will require more running training time than running 5 kilometres or 10 kilometres.

Preparing for the big day

Preparing for the big day starts well before the race. You should have been eating well, with lots of carbohydrates and plenty of variety in your diet all through your training programme. With a week to go you will be tapering your training; that is reducing its volume so that you are fresh for the event. Regardless of the fact that you are running less you should keep your food intake up, concentrating on high carbohydrate foods such as rice, pasta, potatoes, etc. You also need to keep your fluid intake up – drinking plain water is best. On the day itself make sure that you have eaten before the race. Again carbohydrate is important, perhaps in the form of a bowl of cereal or some toast.

You should wear kit and shoes that you have run in before. Don't buy new running kit and new shoes and socks and then keep them for the race. Even though they may look good and feel fine when you try them on in the shop, when you run in them you may find that they rub or cause blisters. Finishing a race with a sore groin where your shorts have rubbed, or your big toe bleeding from a blister is no fun. If you are prone to sore legs, armpits or nipples from chafing of clothing, use a smear of petroleum jelly to lubricate the area before you start.

The start of the race

So the day of the race comes and you are nervous. You will probably visit the toilet more than once before the race. Often toilets at races run out of toilet paper, so it is worth carrying some tissues with you before the start. You need to keep well hydrated. Keep taking water on board as you warm up and stretch. A common mistake for beginners is purposely not to drink before a race so that they won't have to stop part way round to relieve themselves. Women especially are prone to making this mistake, more so if they have any pelvic floor problems. Unfortunately if you start the race dehydrated the whole run will be much more stressful. Dehydration will reduce your blood volume, which will reduce your stroke volume so that your heart will have to beat harder to maintain cardiac output. Your heart rate will already be raised because of the anticipation of the race and your response to being nervous. You may have to register before the start of the race, but even if you don't, try to arrive at least an hour before the start. Wear your kit, and if necessary a tracksuit over the top to keep you warm.

Warm up by gently jogging and gradually increasing the pace. When you are warm, stretch well, leaving your tracksuit on. Warm muscles stretch better than cold ones. Having stretched keep jogging about until you move to the start line. Choose your place on the start line according to the time in which you think you will finish the race. Sometimes race organisers will arrange the start area into finishing times, the fastest people standing right on the start line and the slower people further back. Starting too far forward impedes faster runners and standing too far back causes you to be impeded by slower people.

Having said that, you should be aware that starting too fast will cause a build-up of lactate in your muscles that will not be completely dissipated during the race and will therefore reduce your performance. Starting among slower runners than yourself is a better option than starting among people who are faster than you are.

A very common mistake is to go off too fast at the start of a race. Set off at a very comfortable pace and gradually increase it. At the start of the race there is a mass surge forwards before people gradually string out, when running at your own pace becomes easier.

After you cross the line put extra clothing on and stretch again while your muscles are still warm.

⑥ Cycling

For many people cycling is a cheap means of transport that easily integrates exercise into everyday activities such as travelling to work. For other people cycling is a great way to explore the countryside. Cycling is an excellent activity for improving the heart and lungs, relieving stress and increasing muscular strength and endurance. In addition, with the introduction of studio cycling, we need not be put off even by those cold, wet days through the winter.

Cycling clubs and events have grown in number to accommodate everyone from the serious competitive cyclist to those who cycle occasionally. Cycle routes through the towns and countryside are often waymarked and are available in map and booklet form, and the Sustrans network of cycle routes covering the whole of the UK have now opened over 6500 miles of National Cycle Network, one-third of which is traffic-free and so ideal for new cyclists and for children.

> Sustrans National Cycle Network; Public Information, 35 King St, Bristol, BS1 4DZ.
> 01179 290888 or 01179 268893,
> fax 01179 294173
> http://www.sustrans.org.uk/webcode/home.asp

To be complete, any fitness programme needs a baseline of low-intensity aerobic work. Simply ensuring that you are active for some part of every day, even if that activity takes only ten or fifteen minutes can be a foundation of healthy activity on which to build levels of fitness. Thus cycling to work, to collect the children from school or to go shopping can all form a part of a multi-sport training programme. Whilst many sportspeople view cycling purely as a sport and do not take seriously someone in their working clothes pedalling steadily, nevertheless that person is regularly adding to a fitness programme at a level of intensity that is important, especially in terms of teaching the body to utilise fat as fuel, and yet that most of us ignore or forget. Often sportspeople find it boring to exercise at low intensity, yet cycling to work can add this level in, while also reducing travelling costs and time that can then be set aside in order to train.

Cycle sport

Cycling is not just one but a number of sports. Road racing involves racing and time trialling on the roads; track racing is carried out at specialised tracks around the country; and cyclocross and mountain-bike racing are also competitive forms of cycling, carried out on rough terrain. Within mountain biking, born cross-country and downhill racing form separate events. Trail quest and Polaris include navigation and are orienteering events on bikes.

All these cycling activities have given rise to specific clubs and specific training for their events; however, most clubs will also accommodate enthusiastic participants who, while they may not want to race, are keen to train with others – so don't be put off if you feel that racing may not be for you.

Choosing your bike and choosing the type of cycling that you enjoy go hand in hand. While many people ride mountain bikes on the road and simply for fitness, road bikes are not really robust enough for rough terrain. Road cycling is popular, since once you can ride a bike then you can immediately start to improve your fitness levels and thus your speed and/or the distance you can cycle at a stretch.

> The cyclist touring club and Audax (http://www.aukhawk.uklinux.net/), the long-distance cycling club, are international and have local branches throughout Britain and Europe. They cater for cyclists who want to ride with a group and set themselves challenges but don't want to race. Other cycling clubs cater for competitive road race, track and time-trial cyclists.

Off-road cycling requires more upper body strength and greater balance than road cycling, so you may find that you also have to improve your skill in handling a bike and in overcoming obstacles. You may spend a percentage of your time picking yourself up from the dirt at first and retrying a particular obstacle; however, the rewards are a traffic free environment and access to places unavailable by car. It is likely that you will be unable to cover the same distance off-road that you are able to cover on the road.

Audax rides cover long distances, often hundreds of kilometres, within a specified time frame, and thus can be a good way not only of motivating yourself to ride further but also of meeting other riders.

Choosing your equipment

The most important part of starting to cycle is to get the equipment right. If the bike has the wrong size frame and so doesn't fit you, or is not set up correctly you will be uncomfortable and find controlling the bike difficult. Deciding on a road, mountain, touring or racing bike, rigid frame or front and rear suspension can be like finding your way through a maze. Don't make the mistake of deciding to buy a cheap bike to see if you like the sport. You may not like it simply because you are riding an unsuitable bike. I started mountain biking on a rigid frame bike and as my skill level off-road was so poor found myself sitting in the dirt and covered in bruises on practically every outing. Finally, having dislocated my shoulder, I lost my nerve and kept to the roads, until a cycling friend persuaded me to try a bike with dual suspension. My off-road cycling started again and this time I stayed on the bike far more. The suspension on the bike not only made the ride more comfortable but compensated for my poor technique and allowed me to ride over obstacles that previously had defeated me. In most parts of the country there are bike hire shops, and so it is possible to try out different types of bike and find out which you like.

Buying a bike

A specialised bike shop will be able to advise on what type of bike is most suitable for you and will set it up in the shop to suit you. They will also be able to advise you on clothing, shoes and a helmet. Padded cycle shorts improve the comfort of the ride and a close-fitting cycle jersey reduces wind resistance and wicks away moisture.

Getting started

Even if you are extremely fit aerobically, if you have never cycled before you will find that you need to learn the movement patterns to become efficient, so don't try to do too much too soon. You may also have to learn to use your gears effectively. Using too high a gear causes leg fatigue very quickly. Try to use a gear that allows you to spin the pedals quite fast but without straining. Use smaller gears for going uphill and a higher gears for downhill.

Start out gently to warm up, gradually increasing the workload by pedalling (spinning) faster or using a higher gear. Cool down at the end of the session by gradually slowing down to reduce the workload. Stretch, concentrating on abdominals, pectorals, triceps, trapezius, gluteals, hip flexors, hamstrings, quadriceps, tibialis anterior (shin), gastrocnemius and soleus (calf).

Safety

- To ride safely — the bike — as well as the rider, must be maintained. You should learn to carry out simple repairs and always carry a basic toolkit and a spare inner tube.

- Most serious injuries from cycling accidents involve injury to the head. Always wear a well-fitting cycle helmet off-road as well as on-road.

- Wear bright colours and use lights in poor visibility.

- Follow the Highway Code.

Spinning and turbo training

Indoor cycling has become popular in health and fitness centres as 'spinning classes'.

'Spinning' normally refers, in cycling circles, to spinning the pedals at a fairly high cadence and so keeping the intensity of the workout high from an endurance perspective.

Serious cyclists ride their road bike on a set of rollers that turn under the wheels as the cyclist pedals. To keep upright he or she has to keep the pedals 'spinning'. The advantage of this training method is that it not only improves the cyclist's balance but also trains the body at a high level of endurance and helps to raise the anaerobic threshold.

An alternative to cycling on rollers is to put the bike on a turbo trainer. This is a device that fixes the back wheel onto a drum that provides an adjustable resistance for you to pedal against and so you can simulate hill work or flat riding etc.

More recently spinning classes have become popular in health clubs. In these classes the participants follow the instructions of an instructor and pedal to music on a bike with a fixed wheel. Such classes can provide a useful way to keep fitness levels up for cycling when the weather conditions are miserable and on winter nights; however, do not expect to be able to get straight out of these classes and immediately perform as if you had been training outside all winter , especially if you normally do most of your riding off-road.

7 Swimming

Swimming is an excellent sport, having the potential to maintain or improve the condition of the heart and lungs, and tone both upper and lower body muscles. To swim well requires a high degree of flexibility and regular swimming will help to maintain that flexibility especially in the shoulder area.

Swimming is a valuable sport for maintaining an optimum weight. A person of ten and a half stone swimming front crawl uses about 11 kcalories per minute, so 30 minutes will use up 330 kcalories.

Swimming can be extremely informal or can involve serious training and competition in galas. Most swimming pools have lane swimming sessions set up for serious competitive swimmers and fitness training. The lanes are divided into slow medium and fast. To choose a suitable lane, watch for a while and pick one in which your swimming speed is compatible with that of others. You may find yourself moving from the medium to the slow, or even the fast to the slow, or vice versa, especially if you swim at different session times on different days. Be guided by your capabilities and speed related to the other swimmers rather than by your notion of whether or not you are a good swimmer, or the label on the lane.

Gertrude Caroline Ederle was the first woman to swim across the English Channel. On 6 August, 1926 she set a new time record, swimming from Cap Gris-Nez, France, to Dover, England, a distance of 56 km (35 miles), in 14 hr 31 min.

The equivalent of this in a 25-metre swimming pool would be 2240 lengths and would burn 9581 kcalories.

Lane swimming protocol requires that you swim up one side of the lane and down the other, and that if someone touches your feet with their hand you move over and let them pass.

Many swimming pools also have a club that organises training and galas and provides coaching in swimming technique. One advantage of training with a club is that the exercise/training session is set by the coach, and so how many lengths, which strokes, when to use a pull buoy or float, and what drills to do are all set by the session coach. Swimming with others also adds a social element and may increase your motivation to work hard at the training and complete each full session.

Most swimming galas have events categorised by age and include various master's age categories in all strokes for both women and men. Swimming clubs generally cater for all age groups. Individual club members vary in how serious they are about their swimming training; some who are highly competitive may train five or six days a week, but others might simply swim with the club once or twice a week and never enter a competition. However fit you are, if your technique is poor in the water you will find swimming exhausting and so it is worth getting some coaching in technique.

Equipment

So long as you have a swimming pool available the only equipment that is vital is a swimming costume and towel. For women a cross-back costume is more suitable for training, while men should wear snug-fitting rather than baggy trunks. Both women and men may find that a swimming cap is useful in that it keeps hair out of the eyes and cuts the amount of water running over your face when you lift your head to breathe.

The water in swimming pools is disinfected and this is likely to make your eyes sore. A pair of well-fitting swimming goggles will combat this problem.

Getting started

Setting a goal to swim once a week will get you started. Increase this as soon as you can, bearing in mind your overall training programme.

If you are new to swim training you will almost certainly benefit from some coaching in technique. If you have had a break from swimming you are likely to find it tiring to start with, especially for the upper body. Start out gently, aiming simply to swim for a given length of time. Do not forget to build up gradually, that is, don't jump into the pool and swim hell for leather, but set off at a steady pace and build it up. Leave enough time for a swim-down/cool-down period at the end of your session. Again some early technique training may pay dividends. Swimming well and comfortably is highly dependent on good technique, and as poor technique practised will often become memorised by the nerve pathways and therefore be very difficult to change later, it is better to check out your technique early on, before you get into more serious training involving much repetition.

You may find the Amateur Swimming Association Swimfit initiative helpful in motivating you. Swimfit provides tips on swimming training technique, nutrition and injury prevention advice, and advice on swimming after injury or heart attack and for weight loss. This is a web-based initiative that provides you with an on-line logbook to track distance and time swum on various strokes and to convert this into calories. You can find Swimfit at www.swimfit.com.

As with all your training you need to work at different intensities in order to get the most from swimming training. You may decide to use perceived exertion to achieve this, training at different rates of perceived exertion at different sessions or mixing different intensities within a session. You may decide to use a heart rate monitor; however, remember that because of the water buoyancy and the horizontal position of swimming, your maximum heart rate will be higher than during land-based activities such as running.

The following training sessions are suggested by Robin Brew, international swimming coach and athlete, for those people with limited training time who want to make the most of their sessions.

The 20 min session
300 with 30 sec + 6 × 50 front crawl with 10 sec
200 with 20 sec + 4 × 50 front crawl with 10 sec
100 with 10 sec + 2 × 50 front crawl with 10 sec

The 30 min session
200 with 30 sec rest
100 faster than 50% of the 200 m time with 30 sec rest
50 faster than 50% of the 100 m time with 30 sec rest
Repeat set 3–4 times – try to increase pace on all four sets

The 40 min session
200 + 4 × 50 alternate 2 × 50 drill, 2 × 50 kick with 10 rest
200 pull + 4 × 40 alternate 2 × 50 drill, 2 × 50 kick with 10 rest
150 with 15 sec
6 × 25 with 10 sec
2 × 75 with 20 sec
4 × 25 with 10 sec
3 × 50 with 20 sec
2 × 25 with 10sec
150 – try to go faster than first 150

(From http://www.robinbrewsports.com/articles/htm)

⑧ Walking

Walking improves the condition of heart and lungs and works the muscles of the lower body. As it is a weight-bearing activity it may improve bone density, and being low impact it puts less stress on the joints than do some other forms of exercise.

The activity of 'fitness walking' became very popular in the USA in the mid-1990s, most notably in those states with a 'pleasant' climate.

> At the International Consensus Symposium on Physical Activity Fitness and Health (ICSPAFH) 1992 Claude Bouchard stated 'Favourable morphological, physiological and metabolic changes are engendered by moderate intensity physical activity, particularly when sessions are frequent and of long duration. Dramatic reduction in the risk profile and improvement in the general health of most adults can be expected with, for instance, a daily one hour walk at about 50% of maximum walking speed'.[1]

That fitness walking failed to take off in colder, wetter parts of the world may well be partly owing to the way the activity was marketed. Whatever it was, the fact remains that walking (as opposed to fitness walking or power walking – a technique of walking fast enough to raise the heart rate significantly) remains one of the most popular activities throughout the Western world. This is hardly surprising as it is something that the vast majority can do, and have done – at least a little – all their lives.

Walking is an ideal activity when starting a fitness programme and a thoroughly enjoyable and convenient way of adding to your multi-sport training programme. You need very little specialised equipment, can vary the intensity very easily, get to see your local area, and can walk alone or with friends.

Many people involved in sports do not think of walking as part of their training programme; however, more people walk than participate in any other sport! A review of sports participation by gender in The General Fitness Household Survey, found that the top five sports were participated in as in Table 8.1.

Table 8.1 Participation in top five sports

	Males (%)	Females (%)	Total (%)
Weight training	9	3	**6**
Cycling	15	8	**11**
Yoga and keep fit	7	17	**12**
Swimming	13	16	**15**
Walking	49	41	**45**

(From The General Household Survey 1996–1997)

Different walking activities

Fitness walking/power walking

'Brisk walking for 45 minutes per day, four times per week will result in a fat loss of 18 lbs over a year provided that there are no changes to diet'

Dr James Rippe, The Complete Book Of Fitness Walking

The faster a person walks the more energy is expended. Indeed, continuously increasing walking pace will eventually lead to a point where walking is such hard work that it is easier to break into a run. Walking at that speed will burn more calories than running at the same speed!

Many people walk on a treadmill especially if the weather is poor or if their time to carry out their fitness activity is in the evening and it is cold and dark. Treadmills can be set for speed and gradient and often have preprogrammed routes built in complete with gradients. It is easy to plot progress by using these set routes as time trials.

What to wear

You need to be dressed for the weather. That is if the weather is warm, a T-shirt and shorts, or whatever is comfortable and not restrictive in any way. Sports shops have very good clothing designed to wick away sweat but remain dry. For women a good sports bra should be worn.

In cold weather it is best to wear a number of thin layers rather than one thick one. A close-fitting, long-sleeved, breathable thermal next to the skin and fleece clothing on top works well. Clothing designed for skiing, cycling or hill walking is ideal. You may need a wind shirt, or a fleece made from wind-stopper fabric, and a waterproof, lightweight jacket. A breathable fabric such as Gore-Tex™ is ideal. A bumbag or small rucksack facilitates carrying a drink and any clothing that you may wish to add or remove as you walk.

You can fitness walk in any comfortable trainers or flat shoes. Again, sports shops have trainers designed for fitness walking, though I have found a comfortable pair of racing flats (running shoes designed for racing in) excellent. As walking is a low-impact activity there is no need for a thickly padded midsole. When looking for shoes make sure that they are not built on too stiff a last. They should flex easily in the area of the toe joints. High ankle cuffs are not a good idea as they are likely to interfere in the foot motion once you start walking faster.

Technique
When starting a walking programme concentrate on walking tall, keeping your chin level with the ground and head centred (not tilting back or with chin jutting out). Relax your shoulders down and back and hold your tummy muscles in. Swing your arms naturally and use an easy stride length. Put your heel down first and roll through to the toe.

Walking faster will increase the calories burned. For instance, increasing your pace from 3 to 4 mph will increase calories used per minute by about 50 per cent. Increasing again to 6 mph will almost double the calorific burn. Power walking or fitness walking, involving a slight change in technique, can accommodate increases in pace of this order.

To power walk or fitness walk you should keep your stance fairly upright, holding your stomach in and lifting your chest without arching your back. Keep your shoulders relaxed but bend your elbows and fix them at a 90-degree angle.

Swing your arms front to back and not across your body. On the forward swing do not force the elbows high. Your arms should swing vigorously but naturally. Swinging your arms faster will cause your feet to follow.

Put the heel down first and roll through to the toe, pushing off from the toe behind you. Do not try to increase your stride length; it is more efficient to stride normally but to increase the speed of the strides – that is, more steps per minute.

When starting a walking programme you should consider what type of activity and how much you already do on a regular basis. Start your walking programme just above this level of activity. If your normal level of activity is to walk for ten minutes to and from the station, then start your walking programme at no more than 15 minutes continuous fast walk, or 30-minute intervals of fast and slow walking.

Table 8.2 is a beginner's programme to start walking as a fitness activity.

The programme should be followed by setting out at a comfortable pace and gradually speeding up until you are walking very briskly and are slightly breathless.

Table 8.2 Beginner's walking for fitness programme

	MONDAY	WEDNESDAY	FRIDAY	SUNDAY	weekly total
WEEK 1	15 mins	15 mins	15 mins		45
WEEK 2	15 mins	15 mins	20 mins		50
WEEK 3	20 mins	15 mins	20 mins		55
WEEK 4	20 mins	15 mins	15 mins	15 mins	65
WEEK 5 (easy week)	15 mins	15mins	20 mins		50
WEEK 6	20 mins	15 mins	15 mins	15 mins	65
WEEK 7	15 mins	15 mins	20 mins	20 mins	70
WEEK 8	15 mins	25 mins	15 mins	20 mins	75

Consistency and progression

Once you have started walking, either as a newcomer to a fitness programme or as a newcomer to walking for fitness and as part of a multi-sport training programme, you need to keep the activity going consistently.

Walking fast uses the muscles of the legs and buttocks – those are the anterior tibialis on the front of the lower leg, the calf muscles on the back of the lower leg, hamstrings on the back of the thigh, and gluteals muscles (the buttock muscles). Perhaps surprisingly, even in a very fit person these muscles may ache after a fitness walking session. Training consistently and progressing gradually will allow you to become used to the activity.

One very good way to progress is to add interval training.

Interval training

Interval training involves walking very quickly for a predetermined distance and then slowing down to recover before repeating the process. For instance, on an athletics track, a person may walk 400 metres as fast as possible and then slow right down to allow for recovery for 200 metres before going again. If this process is repeated four times, a set of four intervals has been achieved. The same system can be utilised using lamp-posts as markers; for instance, walk for three lamp-posts briskly and then one slowly; or using a timer, maybe walking for three minutes briskly and three minutes slowly, with repeats.

Hill training

During this type of training the walker should find a gradient of a suitable length and steepness and walk uphill hard, recovering on the way down. As with interval training the process is repeated for a set number of times. Walking uphill raises the intensity dramatically. You should lean into the hill from the ankles rather than bending excessively from the waist, so that your stance remains relatively upright. I find it helpful to focus my eyes near to the top of the hill rather than giving in to the temptation of looking at my feet.

Race walking

Race walking can be highly competitive or sociable and friendly.

At one end of the scale are highly tuned Olympic athletes and at the other are fun race walkers, often to be found holding their own in the middle of a field of fun runners.

If you wish to learn race walking techniques or to enter race walking competitions contact your local athletics club, who will be pleased to help you.

WOMEN'S WORLD RECORDS			
5,000 m 20:17.19	Kerry Saxby AU	Sydney, Australia	14 Jan. 1990
10,000 m 41:56.23	Nadezhda Ryashkina SU	Seattle, Washington, US	24 July 1990

The countryside, hills and fells

There are many opportunities to walk. As with fast walking, walking over hills will improve the fitness of the heart and lungs (cardiovascular system). Rambling, trail-blazing, hill walking and backpacking all use the vast network of footpaths and bridleways found all over the United Kingdom. Some of these footpaths take in the hills and mountaintops, and are quite steep and rough in places. Others take lowland routes through valleys or around coastal clifftops. Exploring these paths may entail getting wet and muddy, but you will find spectacular beauty, picturesque scenery, peace and tranquillity. You could also join a club or group and make your walking a social activity. Rambling and long-distance walking both involve walking in the countryside in groups. The group follows a set route and usually aims to start together and meet up again at the finish, often at a pub. The chosen routes use footpaths and bridleways, waymarked paths, national trails, open spaces, access land, common land and national parks. Long-distance walks are those over 20 miles long and include the long-distance footpaths that are often several hundred miles in length. There are many books, maps, and websites giving details and directions of these walks. Challenge walking involves accomplishing set routes within particular time limits – these routes could be anything between ten and a few hundred miles in distance.

Hill and fell walking refer to walking on fells and mountain areas. Walking up a hill increases the workload and the energy cost considerably; carrying a pack increases it further. Walking downhill also increases the energy cost over walking on the level; however, if you are unaccustomed to downhill walking you will become very sore, as muscles are used eccentrically as shock absorbers.

Orienteering, carried out in the countryside or large parks, is a form of competitive walking (or running). Orienteers use a large scale, minutely detailed map to navigate their way around a pre-set course, finding checkpoints. The object is to visit the checkpoints to complete the course in as short a time as possible. Some orienteers walk the whole distance and some run the whole way but most mix walking and running, depending on their fitness levels and the terrain.

Footwear and clothing in the countryside

In the countryside, especially on the hills, the weather can change dramatically and quickly. If the ground is hilly and rough you will need stout shoes or boots, or fell running shoes, available from any good outdoor activities shop. Walking boots and shoes have moulded grip-giving soles and can be re-waterproofed as necessary. It is best to wear layers of warm but breathable clothing; there are many lightweight thermal garments on the market. It is also a good idea to carry a small rucksack in which to keep any layers you are not wearing, a drink and possibly some snacks.

Building walking into your training programme

While fitness race and hill walking can require high intensity aerobic activity, and so can be fitted into any programme as the aerobic training component, they can also easily be reduced in intensity and thus fit very well into any programme as the lower-intensity, long-duration activity that is important for all-round fitness.

A complete day out walking in the countryside on a fairly regular basis, say once a fortnight or once every three weeks, can add to a training programme considerably, both from a physiological point of view and in terms of motivation and mental, emotional and spiritual health.

In young people strength is generally enough for everyday tasks to be carried out but in the elderly – even healthy elderly – strength and power are often near to or so far below functionally important thresholds that the ability to perform vital everyday tasks,[1] such as getting out of a chair or climbing stairs, is lost. Just to perform basic tasks, such as getting dressed, can result in immense fatigue, comparable to that of the athlete at the limit of their performance capabilities.

> Position statements from the US Surgeon General's Office, based on worldwide research, uphold strength training as a key factor in maintaining functional ability, health and independence as we age.

Muscle strength and power decline with old age even in completely healthy individuals. At every age the strength of a muscle is directly related to its cross sectional area – therefore age-related decline in muscle mass reduces muscle strength and power.[2] Strength is therefore an important part of a multi-sport training programme whether it be strength for health, to improve sport, to improve physique or to balance out aerobic work and flexibility in a general fitness programme

Women – 'the weaker sex'?

For women strength training is extremely important. Women are weaker than men both in absolute terms and in relation to body weight. Their poorer power-to-weight ratio means they are likely to be ten years ahead of men in their loss of ability to perform daily physical tasks. This poorer power-to-weight ratio is reflected in the lower step heights achievable by healthy elderly women[3] and in the greater prevalence of disability and of falls among elderly women than among elderly men.

This advantage can be greatly offset by training for strength and balance. For women involved in sports, poor strength may be reflected in increased risk of injury. While strength training can greatly reduce the risk of injury, many women are afraid to train for strength in case they build a lot of muscle. However, building muscle bulk requires a lot of dedication. Many competitive bodybuilders train for two to three hours a day, five or six days a week; their goal is not to show superior strength but to build muscle mass, and so their training is specifically designed to achieve this goal. Even given this dedication to training, in practice it is very difficult for the majority of women to build large amounts of muscle naturally; that is, without chemical enhancement, as they lack the necessary hormonal stimulus. Thus the chances of becoming over muscled are remote and are outweighed by the benefits of strength training for women.

How should I train for strength?

A strength programme should follow the principle of specificity.

It should be specific to your immediate needs and work towards your long-term goals. Many variables need to be taken into account:

- Which muscle groups should be included?

- Should exercises be compound or isolation?

- What type of muscle action is needed (e.g. isometric, isotonic, concentric, eccentric)?

- What are the predominant energy sources involved in the sport?

- Are there any common injury sites involved?

The programme may be progressed by:

- increasing the number of reps in a set;

- increasing the number of sets;

- increasing the load;

- changing the sets system;

- changing the exercises;

- increasing the number of exercises per part of the body.

What type of resistance should I use?

Many beginners to strength work prefer fixed resistance machines to free weights, and indeed this is all that is available in some clubs and centres. Although fixed resistance machines are arguably easier to learn, a mixture of both free weights and fixed resistance accommodates using lifting techniques that are readily transferable

> ## Rule of thumb
>
> As with other aspects of the multi-sport training programme it is wise to increase only one aspect of the strength programme at a time.
>
> Generally if the number of reps in a set is increased first, dropping the number of reps again can accommodate a subsequent increase in resistance.

to actions common in everyday life and also, when performed well, improve body awareness and control.

When training for sports performance it should be noted that increases in strength gained from weight training may or may not translate to improved performance. Increased strength may be more applicable by adding resistance when performing the sport, for instance increasing the resistance on a rowing ergometer, or using a higher than normal gear on a bike.

Strength for sport

Strength training with weights may not translate into improved sports performance. Much of the initial increase in strength comes from neurogenic changes; that is, one learns to innervate the muscle fibres in the right sequence. To be effective in improving performance strength work needs to mimic closely the action of the sport. For this reason when training for improved sports performance using weights, free weights are preferable because the movement patterns are adaptable, whereas fixed resistance machines set the movement patterns for the lifter.

Working with rubber tubing or rubber bands, or working with a partner may also provide useful resistance modes for sportspeople; however, adding resistance during participation in the sport, so long as that resistance is not so great as to alter technique, may provide the most appropriate training.

Remember that to assist sports performance, strength training has to be specific while also maintaining body balance. The programme should take into account:

- specific muscles used in the sport either as prime movers or fixators;

- joint angles;

- type of contraction;

- type of load;

- the balance between strength and muscular endurance;

- predominant energy source;

- common injury sites;

- previous injury sites.

So is weight training helpful to sports people?

What has been said so far does not mean that weight training is not useful to sportspeople.

Although much strength can be gained without increasing muscle mass simply by improving recruitment of fibres, strength is directly proportional to the cross-sectional area of muscle. If increased strength is desirable then working towards muscle hypertrophy and at the same time working on the skill element of the sport such that one learns to utilise the increased muscle mass may be of help.

In sports that put tremendous stress on particular joint structures, increased strength built in the gym may stabilise the joints and help to prevent injury during participation.

> Increased quadriceps and hamstring strength may stabilise the knees of fell runners running downhill. Increased strength and muscle mass may stabilise the shoulder girdle and cervical spine of rugby players in a scrum.

When do I do my strength training?

Strength training for general fitness or health can take place all the year round; however, when training for sports performance the increased stress of the competitive season should be accommodated. This can be done using periodisation or organising appropriate training cycles. An athlete in the competitive season needs to peak for performance and cannot put too much energy into a heavy weight training programme at that time. Substantial amounts of strength work can, however, be built into the off-season in preparation for competition the following year.

Order of exercises

The order of strength exercises may be governed partly by the sets system being used. For instance a superset system requires opposing muscle groups to be worked in sequence. Generally speaking it is advisable to work the largest muscle groups first, using compound exercises, and the muscles of the trunk (abdominal muscles and erector spinae) last. This ensures that these important muscles are not then fatigued before being used to stabilise the spine during other lifts.

Table 9.1 Order of strength exercises

	Back	Chest	Legs	Shoulders and arms	Abdominal exercises
Major muscle group (compound) exercises	chins lat pulldown pullovers single arm row seated pulley row deadlift (lower back)	flat bench press inclined bench press press-ups	deadlift squats lunges step-ups	shoulder press upright row	abdominal curls crunches reverse abdominal curls pelvic tilts oblique curls circle crunches
Isolation exercises	dorsal raise sand lizard	dumbell flyes pec dec	leg extension leg curls	lateral raise bicep curl preacher curl dumbell screw curl tricep extension tricep pushdown tricep kickback bent over flyes	

How many repetitions and sets do I do?

Weight training is usually carried out in sets and reps (repetitions). One rep is the performance of the lift once. A set is a predetermined number of repetitions. Each set may be performed one or more times, i.e. one, two, three or more sets. Different combinations of sets have different terms attached to them. Each individual time a movement is completed is a repetition. A number of repetitions together comprises a set. Strength training adaptations are slightly different, depending on the load and the number of sets and reps used. Three sets of ten reps per exercise are common; however, load, number of reps per exercise and rest between sets should be adjusted according to whether the emphasis is for strength or for endurance: a low number of reps with a heavier load and longer rest favours strength; a high number of reps with a lighter load and shorter rest period favours endurance. It may be that the goal will change as the body adapts. For instance, it may be advisable to build strength first and then start to increase reps and reduce rest in order to add endurance.

How much weight should I lift?

Before you start, predetermine the number of reps to be used in each set and the weight that you are going to lift. To maximise progression you should use the greatest resistance with which you can carry out the lift safely. Thus you should find your repetitions maximum (RM).

Your RM is the greatest resistance that you can overcome for a particular lift. Thus the heaviest weight that can be lifted for ten reps (i.e. an eleventh is not possible) is known as 10 repetitions maximum (ten reps max or 10RM). The heaviest weight that can be lifted for six repetitions is known as 6RM. The maximum for one repetition would be 1RM.

How do I find my repetition maximum?

When beginning a weight training programme you should work well within your capabilities for each lift. However, as you progress, in order to gain maximum benefits you will need to start overloading by using your personal RM for the number of repetitions in your set. To find your RM decide on the number of reps needed and then load the machine (or bar) to a level that you think you can handle. Try for the number of reps you have decided on. If that was too easy, try again with more resistance. If you didn't complete the stated number of reps then drop the resistance lower.

> **Spotters**
> A spotter is there to help you. He or she should hand you the bar or dumbells when necessary and should stay with you to help out if you start to fail. Also he or she can take the bar or dumbells again at the end of your lift.

This trial and error method is hard work. Make sure that you have an experienced lifter with you to spot for you and encourage you. The **spotter** needs to be in a position to take the weight should you fail in your attempt to lift it. If you work out your RM for each lift in your programme all in one session you will have had a good workout. Don't attempt a further workout on the same day.

Sets systems

For newcomers to weight training, each weights workout should use a whole-body approach, covering all the major muscle groups and working with compound exercises that is, exercises that use large muscle groups and utilise more than one muscle.

Simple circuits

A useful starting point is the simple circuit. This will enable you to utilise the whole body in a series of lifts and so to practise your technique without overtraining.

Newcomers to lifting should use a resistance that is within their capabilities rather than trying for RM. The simple circuit involves completing one set of each exercise performed. A programme may then read as in Table 9.2. One or more circuits may be performed, depending on your fitness level.

Basic sets

In basic sets each set is repeated for the desired number of times (e.g. 3 sets), resting for a short period in between each set, as in Table 9.3. This system is used with less resistance than the RM and is therefore also suitable when working on a maintenance programme. The amount of weight used should be such that you can complete all three sets of ten, although the third set is hard work.

Table 9.2 Simple circuit programme

Exercise	Reps
deadlift	10
bench press	10
lunges	10
lat pulldown	10
squats	10
alternate dumbell press	10
abdominal curls	10
dorsal raise	10

Table 9.3 Basic sets

Exercise	Reps
deadlift	10 × 3
bench press	10 × 3
lunges	10 × 3
lat pulldown	10 × 3
squats	10 × 3 etc.

Delorme sets

In this system the RM is halved for the first set. For the second set three-quarters of the RM is used, and for the third set the full amount is used (see Table 9.4).

Table 9.4 Delorme sets (where 10RM for the squat is 60 kilos)

First set	30 k × 10
Second set	45 k × 10
Third set	60 k × 10

Rest is allowed between each set, and failure to complete the final set may occur. Because of this it is a good idea to have a spotter on hand especially if working with free weights.

Simple sets

In this system the RM is used for each set and it is accepted that the lifter may fail to reach the predetermined number of repetitions towards the end of the sets. Thus the number of repetitions will automatically be reduced after the first set, despite the fact that the lifter is still aiming for the full number (see Table 9.5). Once three sets of ten can be performed at 40 kilos then the resistance is increased. In this system, each set is performed to failure.

Table 9.5 Simple sets (where 10RM for the bench press is 40 kilos)

First set	40 k × 10
Second set	44 k × 8 (still aiming for 10)
Third set	40 k × 6 (still aiming for 10)

Advanced set systems

There are many other sets systems, some of which were developed for strength or physique athletes and aim to develop these attributes to the limit of the individual's genetic potential. The systems outlined above are good basic lifting systems that can be used for development of muscular strength or endurance.

To train for absolute strength the lifter should use high resistance and low reps, for instance, 6RM. To train for muscular endurance the lifter should use less resistance but more reps – up to 20RM.

⑩ Flexibility

'I never was naturally flexible and no matter what I do I cannot touch my toes'

An important area of any training programme is training for flexibility. Flexibility is important for health in maintaining freedom of movement as we age, and important in sports performance in maintaining range of movement.

> Flexibility is joint-specific. A person with great shoulder flexibility, who can easily do up a zip at the back of the neck, may be totally unable to touch his or her toes without bending the knees.

The method used to measure flexibility is reflected by flexibility scores and should be taken into account. For instance ability to touch the toes while keeping the legs straight is affected by degree of flexion at the hip joint and the joints of the lower back, length of the hamstrings, and indeed length of the legs in comparison to that of the torso and arms and size of the abdomen. However, being able to touch one's toes is commonly used as a measure of hamstring flexibility. Whilst hamstring flexibility does affect this movement being unable to touch one's toes while keeping the legs straight may simply reflect long legs in relation to the torso.

No matter what we do to measure flexibility, ease of movement keeps us looking and feeling younger, and it is possible to improve or maintain flexibility by using full range of movement exercises and by stretching.

Should I stretch my tendons or my muscles?

Within and around the muscle tissues is connective tissue, the endomysium, perimysium and the ectomysium. This connective tissue is made up of elastin and collagen, the collagen being resistant to stretch. The genetically decided structure of the connective tissue, in terms of how much collagen there is in relation to how much elastin, has an effect on natural flexibility. If we are born with more collagen then we will be less flexible, whereas more elastin makes us more flexible. When we talk about stretching we almost always talk about stretching the muscle; however, in practice, it is actually the connective tissue within the muscle belly, not the protein element of the muscle, which is resistant to stretch and which we try to affect.

Active range of movement

The active range of movement (ROM) is the range of movement when only the muscles affecting that movement are used. Thus to measure active flexion at the hip a person would be asked to lift one leg up in front of them as far as possible, using only their own muscle power, and the degree of hip flexion achieved simply by contracting the hip flexor muscles would be measured.

As the hip flexors are contracting to lift the leg, tension in the opposing muscle group, the hip extensors (hamstrings and gluteal muscles), causes resistance to hip flexion. The less flexible the hip extensors are the more resistance they provide and thus the greater the strength that is required to flex the hip.

Sport and flexibility

Clearly then, active ROM is affected not only by the degree of flexibility of the opposing muscle group, the **antagonist muscles**, but also the strength of the muscle group responsible for the movement, the **agonist**. Active hip flexion in ballet dancers is often remarkable, demonstrating superior strength as well as superior flexibility as they lift a perfectly straight leg to shoulder height and smile sweetly.

Muscles work in pairs.

The muscle contracting to affect the movement is called the **agonist**.

The muscle opposite that, which has to relax in order for movement to happen, is called the **antagonist**.

Active range of movement is important in many sports, especially diving, gymnastics, swimming, rock climbing, sprinting, Olympic weightlifting and competitive bodybuilding.

Passive range of movement

Passive ROM is demonstrated when joint movement is assisted by an outside force, as would occur if someone else were to lift a person's leg up in front of them in order to measure passive hip flexion. The outside force may be another muscle group, as when we wrap a towel around our feet and pull on it with our arms in order to stretch the hamstrings; or it may be gravity, as in standing straight-legged touching our toes, or it may be another outside influence, another person for instance, helping us as in partner stretches.

Age and flexibility

An inactive adult loses about five to seven pounds of muscle every decade. Therefore an inactive 50-year-old has about 15–20 lb less muscle than when he or she was 20[1], with a consequential decrease in the ability to produce force. This results in the muscle groups of the lower limb in a 70-year-old being able to produce approximately just 60 per cent of the force generated by young adults.[2] This loss of muscle mass, known as sarcopenia, can be seen as a reduction in the number of muscle fibres. As we age we lose the contractile elements of the muscle and more collagen is laid down in their place, so the muscles become more resistant to stretch and we become less flexible. Added to this the opposing muscle groups lose power and exacerbate the loss of range of movement. Unless we work on flexibility and strength as we age we stiffen up.

Stretching

When should I stretch?

Much research has been done investigating when is a good time to stretch. Most people agree that a short stretch period should be built in to the warm-up session to ensure that the joints have been through the full range of movement that they will be required to use during the activity. This is best performed as active stretching, the range of movement being gradually increased as the muscle tissue warms up.

Other than that a stretch period is generally agreed to be useful at the end of the activity to ensure that muscles are returned to their normal resting length. Increases in flexibility however are most probably more likely to occur when the muscle is not fatigued. Separate stretching sessions lasting from anywhere between 10 minutes and a half an hour can be built into the multi-sport training programme (always remember to stretch only warm muscle).

Some research shows that the more often we stretch the more effective it is. Utilising a few minutes at odd times during the day to stretch can therefore be very beneficial.

How should I stretch?

We may improve flexibility using active or passive stretching, ballistic or static stretching or combinations of these.

Active stretching

When we stretch using an active ROM, it is known as 'active stretching'. That is, we use one muscle group's contraction to put the joint through a range of movement that stretches the opposing muscle group. Sitting or standing upright and pulling the shoulder blades together by contracting the muscles of the upper back stretches the muscles of the chest. This is an active stretch.

Ballistic stretching

Often this type of stretching involves bouncing at the end of the ROM or ballistic stretching. Kicking the legs up in the air in front of you as in the can-can is a ballistic stretch. Straight-legged toe touching and bouncing downwards towards the floor is a ballistic stretch. Whilst undoubtedly effective in improving flexibility, ballistic stretching carries with it a high risk of damage to the muscle or joint.

> **Active stretching** without ballistic movement is a very effective way of simultaneously increasing flexibility and strength specific to active ROM.

Passive stretching

Passive stretching involves an outside influence moving the limb and so taking the joint through to the end of its range of movement. Sitting on the floor with a towel or belt around your feet and pulling the body forwards towards the thighs stretches the hamstrings and lower back passively. Lying on your back while a partner lifts your straight leg up into the air and through to the end of your range of flexion also involves passive stretching. This does not require strength from the opposing muscle group.

Static stretching

Static stretching occurs when the joint is moved slowly towards the end of the ROM and held still. This type of stretching carries with it less risk of injury than does ballistic stretching.

Stretch reflex

When a muscle is stretched nerve receptors situated in the muscle cells set off a nervous reflex causing that same muscle to contract and oppose the stretch. The faster the stretch movement the stronger the contraction will be. This is known as the stretch reflex or myotatic reflex and acts as a safety mechanism. As the joint moves towards the end of its ROM the risk of injury to joint structures and soft tissues increases, thus in order to prevent this the muscle contracts and moves the joint back towards neutral and away from the end of its range.

If we move slowly into the stretch until we feel resistance from the muscle, and at that point hold the position still (static stretch), the stretch reflex will be overcome and the muscle will again relax, allowing us to move further into the stretch, which should be done slowly.

Golgi tendon organ reflex

Golgi tendon organs (GTOs) are nerve receptors located within the tendons. Putting tension on a tendon, as may occur during stretch but more often occurs during a muscle contraction, may fire the Golgi tendon organ reflex causing the muscle to relax. The GTOs sense that the tendon is under tension and therefore in a precarious position and so they fire, setting off a reflex relaxation in the muscle in order to release tension on the tendon.

This particular reflex facilitates an advanced method of stretching called peripheral neuromuscular facilitation, more commonly known as PNF.

Peripheral neuromuscular facilitation (PNF)

PNF stretching utilises the GTO reflex by purposely putting the tendon under tension, thus causing the reflex action of muscle relaxation.

To use PNF stretching, move slowly into the stretch position until you feel the muscle is extended; wait for the stretch reflex to be overcome and at that point move further into the stretch position until the muscle is under tension. Holding this position, contract the muscle hard isometrically, that is, contract or tense the muscle without any movement occurring at the joints and hold this contraction for 6–10 seconds.[3] This will put tension on the tendons and fire the GTOs. Now relax the muscle and wait for a few seconds until the muscle will allow you to move (slowly) further into the stretch.

CRAC

CRAC stretching is a combination of active stretching and PNF stretching. Muscles work in pairs, an agonist and an antagonist. As one muscle contracts, its antagonist relaxes to allow movement around a joint to occur. This is known as reciprocal innervation.

To use CRAC follow the PNF method of stretching:

• Move slowly into the stretch position, waiting for the stretch reflex to be overcome in the antagonist.

• **C**ontract the muscle hard isometrically for 6–10 seconds.

• Now **R**elax the muscle and wait for a few seconds.

• **A**ctively **C**ontract the agonist to move (slowly) further into the stretch.

> **C**ontract
> **R**elax
> **A**ctively
> **C**ontract

• As you actively contract the agonist, reciprocal innervation will cause the antagonist to relax even further.

To stretch the hamstrings by this method:

• Lie on your back on the floor and raise one straight leg leaving the other leg bent at the knee and foot flat on the ground.

• Holding behind the leg with your hands or a towel move slowly to stretch the hamstrings and wait for the muscle to relax.

• Now contract the hamstrings hard for 6–10 seconds by pushing the leg down towards the ground, against the towel, but do not let the leg move.

• Relax the muscle.

• Contract the hip flexors to move the leg towards your chest and further into the stretch.

This method of stretching is very effective in increasing active range of movement as it simultaneously stretches one muscle while strengthening the opposite muscle.

Is stretching ever bad for me?

If you have lax ligaments around a joint you may have a hypermobile joint. In this case strengthening the muscles to stabilise the joint and protect it from injury is more appropriate than stretching these muscles.

Muscles that are sore from being overworked should not be stretched until the soreness dissipates.

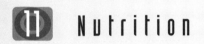

To move we must utilise energy, and to replace the energy we use we must eat. Also, by virtue of the fact that when we train to overload, as we must do if we are to benefit from improved fitness, the training causes damage to the muscles and puts extra strain on the body systems in general, so we need to rebuild and repair. If we have broken down the body tissues with training we need to feed them the right ingredients so that they will be stronger after repair and more able to cope. If we fail to eat well then we are more likely to become ill or injured. Good nutrition is the perfect partner to a good training programme.

> 'There is evidence that the number of injuries that occur, as well as the extent of muscle damage, is greater in people who exercise with low muscle glycogen levels. When glycogen stores are depleted, co-ordination is likely to be impaired. This may, in part, explain the increased injury rate.'[1]
>
> *Ronald Maughan, Ph.D.*
> *University Medical School, Foresterhill, Aberdeen, Scotland*[1]

What do I need to eat?

A balance of nutrients is important for both health and fitness training. In relation to some nutrients, such as minerals and vitamins, the body will continue to function reasonably normally for a short while even with an imbalance in the diet, though eventually the imbalance will make itself known. In the case of other nutrients, such as carbohydrates and water, the effects of deficiency are of acute onset. For the active individual a basic understanding of good nutritional principles is therefore vital.

The balanced diet

To obtain a healthy balance of carbohydrates, fats and proteins and to ensure adequate intake of vitamins, minerals and trace elements we should attempt to eat more starchy carbohydrate foods such as bread, cereals and rice, more fresh fruit and vegetables and less fatty foods. The US Department of Health and Human Service published a food pyramid which depicts a base of starchy foods and suggests that oils, fats and sweets should be used sparingly.

However many calories you consume in a day, the balance of foodstuffs within that calorie allowance should remain the same, with most calories coming from complex carbohydrate foods.

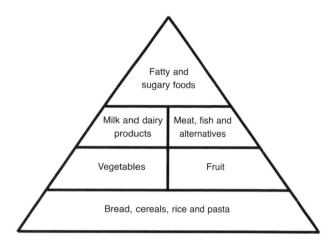

Figure 11.1 Food pyramid as guide to nutrition

For most generally active individuals a well-balanced diet following the guidelines in this chapter will be adequate for whatever activity that they do. For those people training more seriously, either for an extreme challenge or for a competitive event, more careful attention to the food they eat is advantageous.

Protein

Protein comes from both animal and vegetable sources and is made up of amino acids, which are often thought of as the building blocks of the body. Amino acids are rather like the letters of the alphabet: by putting them together in various sequences we can make words, or in the case of amino acids, by putting them together in various sequences we can make different proteins. Protein is found in hormones, enzymes, blood and all body tissues, thus it is very important to us.

In the alphabet there are five vowels. As any one who has played Scrabble will know, without these vowels we cannot make words. In the alphabet of amino acids there are eight essential amino acids without which we cannot make proteins. All eight of the essential amino acids are found in animal proteins such as milk, eggs, cheese and meats. However, to achieve a full complement of essential amino acids from vegetable sources we need to vary our protein sources by mixing grains with pulses or with nuts. Therefore grains such as bread, rice, and pasta can be mixed with beans and legumes or with nuts and seeds in order to reach a full amino acid complement.

Fats

Many people mistakenly think that they should cut out fat from their diet completely. However the body needs fats as a valuable source of energy, to supply and store the fat soluble vitamins, A, D, E and K, and to supply essential fatty acids without which we cannot function healthily.

Because fat makes food palatable and fills us up we add it to all sorts of Western refined foodstuffs, and the result is often a diet too rich in fat. This type of diet has

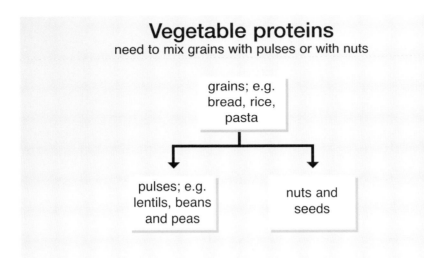

Figure 11.2 Vegetable proteins

been linked to increased levels of obesity and disease, with the result that we in the Western world are encouraged to reduce the amount of fat in our diets.

> We still need some fat in our diets, though recommendations are that to remain healthy no more than 33 pee cent of our calories should come from fat.

Carbohydrates

Carbohydrate foods, often described as the sugary and starchy foods, are the main source of energy for all activities. If carbohydrate intake is low then the levels of glucose in the blood drop and muscle glycogen levels become depleted. Carbohydrate is the only energy source for the brain and central nervous system. Low blood glucose levels affect the ability to concentrate and there is evidence that when carbohydrate intake is low co-ordination is impaired and accidents and injuries occur more frequently.

When blood glucose levels drop we start to feel irritable, weak, shaky and unable to concentrate. Tests also show that reaction time is impaired when carbohydrate levels are low.

How much of each should I eat?

Guidelines vary from country to country and year to year but generally health guidelines agree that for an active individual the proportions of fat, carbohydrate and protein eaten should be divided by the kcals that they supply. Not more than 33 per cent of kcals should come from fat; 10–15 per cent of kcals should come from protein and the remaining 55–60 per cent of kcals should come from carbohydrate sources.

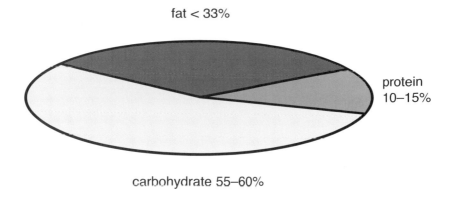

fat < 33%

protein
10–15%

carbohydrate 55–60%

Figure 11.3 Guide to balance of kcals

How do I know how many kcals I consume from each?

Foods supply different amounts of energy per gram dependent on the make-up of the food. Fat is very energy-dense and supplies about 9 kcals per gram. Protein and carbohydrate each supply around 4 kcals per gram. So to work out how many kcals in a particular food come from fat, from carbohydrate or from protein, simply multiply the total number of grams by the energy from that foodstuff.

That is: if a food is made up of 20 grams of fat, 60 grams of carbohydrate and 20 grams of protein and has 500 kcals per 100 grams then

20 grams of fat = 20 × 9 kcals = 180 kcals
180 ÷ 360 × 100 = 36
Therefore in this foodstuff 36% of the kcals come from fat.

20 grams of protein = 20 × 4 kcals = 80 kcals
80 ÷ 360 × 100 = 16
Therefore in this foodstuff 16% of the kcals come from protein.

60 grams of carbohydrate = 60 × 4 kcals =240 kcals
240 ÷ 360 × 100 = 48
Therefore in this foodstuff 48% of the kcals come from carbohydrate.

Overall in your diet you should eat foods that are less than 33 per cent fat and have a high carbohydrate content.

Of course, if you work all of this out for everything you eat you have no time left for training, therefore simply following the food pyramid and being a little stricter on your fat consumption and enjoying eating complex carbohydrates and vegetables should suffice to balance your diet while still leaving you with plenty of time to train.

Weight loss

A very simple formula should help us with this apparently complex area (see box). Calorie requirements are different for everyone dependent on their genetics, age,

Calories in > calories out = weight gain
Calories out > calories in = weight loss

gender, lean body mass, and current activity level. To lose weight we must expend more calories in daily living and in activity than we take in as food. Put simply, to lose weight we must eat less, exercise more, or better still a mixture of both.

To lose 1 lb in weight, we need to create an energy deficit of 3,500 calories. Over a week that amounts to creating an energy deficit of 500 calories per day. That means we can eat 500 calories

3,500 calories ÷ 7 days per week = 500 calories per day.

less per day in order to lose 1 lb of weight per week. However, by combining diet and exercise we could lose the same amount of weight by eating just 250 calories less and expending 250 calories in exercise per day.

Attempting to lose more weight than 1–2 lb a week is not advised. Where more weight loss than this occurs it is often due to loss of muscle mass as well as fat mass.

Severe calorie restriction

- low muscle glycogen levels and low blood glucose levels predispose the athlete to fatigue and injury.
- Weight loss is in part due to glycogen and associated water loss.
- Fatigue makes it difficult to increase energy expenditure.
- The body breaks down muscle to fuel the energy needs.

When calorie restriction is severe the resultant deficit in carbohydrate intake causes low muscle glycogen levels and low blood glucose levels, predisposing the athlete to fatigue and injury. Also carbohydrate is always stored alongside water, one molecule of carbohydrate with three molecules of water, thus some of the apparent weight loss that occurs with severe calorie restriction is due to glycogen and associated water loss, rather than to fat loss. In addition the low glycogen levels cause fatigue, with the result that it is difficult to increase energy expenditure through training.

Finally, during severe calorie restriction exercise is partially fuelled with protein, taken from broken down muscle, so that some of the weight loss is of muscle rather than fat.

Weight loss and multi-sport training

When we train for single-sport events we are limited to how much repetition the body can take before overuse injuries start to occur. By multi-sport training we can increase energy expenditure by training for longer duration or more often, without subjecting the body to the same risk of overuse injuries.

More about carbohydrates

Carbohydrate is needed in order to utilise fat as fuel. In prolonged endurance activity when carbohydrate levels are depleted we start to fuel the exercise by breaking down our body proteins. We use our own muscle to fuel the exercise. Thus carbohydrate is protein-sparing. The greater the carbohydrate stores the less likely we are to use muscle protein to fuel long-duration exercise. The amount of glycogen stored in the muscles is directly related to dietary carbohydrate intake; however, even a well-nourished human being can only store about 1500 to 2000

Rule of thumb
Base your meals around carbohydrates rather than proteins. Think, what carbohydrate am I going to eat, will it be bread, rice, pasta? Now what vegetables shall I put with it? Finally what protein shall I add?

kcals of carbohydrate. We therefore need to replace our carbohydrate stores regularly by ensuring that a large percentage of the calories we consume come from carbohydrate foods. In most Western diets only about 40 per cent of the total kcals are obtained from carbohydrate sources, yet recommendations for athletes are that 70 per cent of the calories should be obtained from carbohydrate.

Studies show that for athletes training one to two hours a day the muscle glycogen levels drop dramatically over a week if carbohydrate intake is normal – that is – around 40 per cent, but glycogen stores drop much less on a high carbohydrate diet.

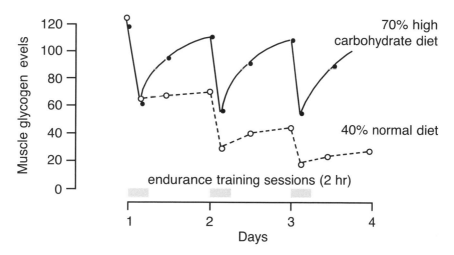

Figure 11.4 Diagram showing the reduction in muscle glycogen levels when endurance training every day on a high carbohydrate diet and on a normal diet (no more than 40% kcals obtained from carbohydrate).

It is advantageous to refuel with carbohydrate immediately after exercise. At this time the muscle is particularly receptive to taking on glycogen and super-compensates, increasing the amount of glycogen stored. For this reason it is recommended that you should eat at least 1.5 grams of carbohydrate per kilogram of body weight within 30 minutes of completing exercise. Thus a 70-kilogram person should eat at least 105 grams of carbohydrate within 30 minutes of stopping exercise. This could be two bananas and three sweet biscuits, or a potato and baked beans. Naturally, as water is taken in to the muscle along with carbohydrate, the athlete should also remain fully hydrated.

Glycaemic Index

In what form you ingest carbohydrate makes a difference to how quickly it is synthesised in the body. Carbohydrates can be classed by Glycaemic Index (GI), those that score high on the glycaemic index being absorbed quickly and those with a low score more slowly. It is thought that eating foods with a low score 30–60 minutes before exercise may maintain a higher blood sugar level at the start of exercise and increase the concentration of fatty acids in the blood, thus improving fat oxidation and reducing reliance on carbohydrate to fuel the exercise. After exercise eating high-scoring foods may restore muscle glycogen more efficiently.

Table 11.1 Glycaemic Index

High Food	Amount for 50 gram of COH
sucrose	50 g
honey	67 g
maple syrup	80 g
bread	4 slices (1" or 28 g each)
breadsticks	7 sticks
wholewheat sweet biscuits	3 biscuits
cornflakes	59 g
muesli	6 tablespoons (70 g)
shredded wheat	3 pieces
Weetabix	4 pieces
raisins	78 g
banana	2 (120 g each)
potato (baked)	1 potato (200 g)
potato (boiled)	254 g
sweetcorn	219 g

Table 11.1 continued...

Moderate Food	Amount for 50 gram of COH
spaghetti;	
macaroni	198 g cooked
noodles	370 g cooked
whole grain rye bread	4 slices (1" each)
rice (white)	169 g cooked
grapes	323 g
orange (navel)	3 oranges (140 g each)
yams (boiled or baked)	168 g
baked beans	485 g
Low food	**Amount for 50 gram of COH**
apple	2.5 (138 g each)
cherries	44 cherries
dates	8 dates
figs	5 figs (fresh, 50 g each)
grapefruit	2.5 (118 g each)
peach	5 (90 g each)
pear	2 (166 g each)
plum	5.5 (66 g each)
butterbeans	292 g
kidney beans	220 g
chickpeas	305 g
grean beans	630 g
green peas	345 g
red lentils	294 g
skimmmed milk	995 ml
yoghurt	658 ml

Table adapted from *The Complete Book of Sports Nutrition* by Anita Bean.

For long-endurance events lasting several hours, such as iron man triathlon, mountain marathon or challenge events, and for stop-and-go sports run as all-day or multi-day tournaments, the athlete should refuel with carbohydrates during the event or between games in the tournament. Again for this purpose carbohydrates with a high to moderate score on the Glycaemic Index are useful.

Fats

Fat is a vital part of hormones, of the insulation around nerve fibres and around vital organs and of cell membranes. Deficiency in certain fatty acids causes ill health.

Fats are made up of high-density lipoproteins (HDL), low-density lipoproteins (LDL) and very low-density lipoproteins (VLDL). Low-density lipoproteins and very low-density lipoproteins are largely found in animal fats and are solid at room temperature. High-density lipoproteins are largely found in vegetable fats and are liquid at room temperature. High total dietary fat intake is a risk factor for coronary heart disease; further, high dietary intake of low-density lipoproteins within a moderate total fat intake is detrimental to health, so wherever possible fat from vegetable sources should be utilised in preference to animal fats.

Fat as fuel

Fat is very energy-dense and as such is a useful fuel. About 50,000–60,000 kcal of energy are stored as fat in the adipose tissue of the body.

Fat is made up of fatty acids and glycerol stored as triglyceride. As well as being stored in the adipose tissue, triglyceride is stored as tiny droplets actually in the muscle fibres. This is known as intramuscular triglyceride. Intramuscular triglyceride provides 2000–3000 kcal of stored energy, far more energy than is stored as muscle glycogen.

Both triglyceride from adipose tissue and intramuscular triglyceride is oxidised to provide energy. As exercise intensity increases from low to moderate intensity the rate of fat oxidation from adipose tissue declines, but due to a relatively large use of intramuscular triglyceride the rate of total fat oxidation increases. Endurance training increases the body's ability to utilise intramuscular triglyceride as fuel.

In comparison to carbohydrate stored as muscle glycogen, fat stores are mobilised and oxidised at relatively slow rates during exercise.

The fat burning myth

At 25 per cent VO_2max, almost all the energy expenditure during exercise is fuelled by fat, whereas at 65 per cent VO_2max only 50 per cent of energy expenditure is fuelled by fat. It is therefore often assumed that the intensity of exercise must be kept low in order to burn fat. However, expressing energy derived from fat as a percentage of energy expenditure without considering total energy expenditure is misleading. Because the total rate of energy expenditure is greater at 65 per cent VO_2max, the absolute rate of fat oxidation is greater than at 25 per cent VO_2max.

Ultimately, reduction of body fat as a result of long-term exercise depends on the total daily energy expenditure and the total daily energy input, rather than on the actual fuel oxidised during exercise.

Calcium, iron and the female athlete

Many female endurance athletes reduce their calorie intake in an attempt to keep their body weight down. Some do not eat enough to meet the Recommended Dietary Allowance of calories for inactive women their age. Low caloric intake is often associated with reduced levels of vitamins and minerals in the diet, thus female athletes who compromise their nutritional status in this way may be deficient in vital nutrients.

One such nutrient that female athletes may be deficient in is calcium. As ready sources of calcium such as milk and cheese also have a high fat content, athletes concerned about their weight may cut out these foods. Low calcium levels are associated with stress fractures and with osteoporosis or brittle-bone disease. Calcium levels should be maintained by eating calcium-rich foods and, where a reduction in fat intake is desirable, using low-fat dairy products.

Because of menstrual blood loss, inadequate diet may also lead to poor iron levels, iron-deficient anaemia and consequently poor performance in endurance sports where the oxygen-carrying capacity of the blood is compromised.

How much do I need to drink?

About 60 per cent of our body weight is made up of water; yet even at rest, through evaporation from the skin and respiratory tract and through excretion, we lose about 2.3 litres of fluid per day.

> During heavy exercise in heat that fluid loss may reach 2–3 litres per hour![2]

Unless we make concerted efforts to replace fluid loss whilst exercising we will become dehydrated. Even slight dehydration is detrimental to performance. For each litre of water lost, heart rate is elevated by about eight beats per minute, cardiac output declines by 1 L/min, and core body temperature rises by 0.3°C. Studies have shown that even a 2 per cent dehydration, when measured by body weight, decreases performance by 6–7 per cent.[3] Dehydration of about 4 per cent will produce a decline in performance of 20–30 per cent!

Drink before you exercise

Despite evidence supporting the need to start exercise well hydrated, many people start training in a dehydrated state.

However, it takes a concerted effort as is not generally usual to drink this much fluid even prior to exercise. In addition many people think about taking on fluid only if they are going to exercise in the heat or if the exercise is going to be intense. Yet fluid loss enough to affect performance occurs even in a cold environment, and many studies show that during long-duration, low- to moderate-intensity exercise such as walking, dehydration is a limiting factor and affects both performance and rate of perceived exertion.

Drink during exercise

Having made the effort to hydrate prior to exercise it is important that during

Limiting factors

In physiological terms there can only ever be one limiting factor to performance. Dependent on the runner's training status, a different physiological adaptation is needed in order to improve performance. Beginners to running will make huge improvements by increasing their cardiac output and thus their MVO_2. However, an athlete who is training regularly may be limited by cellular adaptations and may make further improvements by increasing the number and size of the capillaries supplying the working muscle and of the mitochondria in the muscle fibres. Thus whereas the beginner may well benefit from doing most training between 60 and 75 per cent of maximum heart rate (MHR) a more advanced runner will benefit from varying the training intensities more. Physiological adaptations run along a continuum from low-intensity to high-intensity training. Where on the training continuum those physiological changes take place is partly dependent on the genetic inheritance and partly on the training status of the athlete. For instance training at a heart rate equal to 85 per cent of MVO_2 will for one athlete be right on the limit of the anaerobic threshold and for another below anaerobic threshold. To reach their potential most athletes will have to so some training at all levels. How much training is spent at different intensities depends on the demands of the sport and the limiting factors in the athlete's performance.

> For deconditioned individuals, training at 60 per cent MVO_2 may be crossing the anaerobic threshold.

Note the adaptations taking place during training are complex and multifaceted. Table 12.1 suggests towards which end of the continuum between low intensity and high intensity (1) different energy systems predominate, (2) fibre type recruitment takes place, and (3) adaptations may be assumed to occur.

The combination of intensity and duration of the stimulus placed upon skeletal muscle fibre changes the metabolic adaptations within them. For instance, sprinting relies on fast twitch fibres and on the anaerobic energy systems. Short sprint bursts, lasting less than 10 seconds but at maximal power, rely heavily on the creatine phosphate (PCr) system and on the high velocity of contraction of type IIB fibres. Lactic acid build-up interferes with the creatine phosphate system, and during training for sprint events the athletes aim to produce maximal power without building up lactic acid. They produce repeats of maximum effort for very short duration. This training may involve work intervals of maximum effort for 5–15 seconds followed by a long recovery period of 1–2 minutes such that the creatine

Table 12.1 Predominate energy systems, fibre type recruitment and adaptions during high and low intensity activity.

	% MVO_2	%MHR	Adaptations	Energy Systems	Fibre type Recruitment
low intensity				Aerobic	Slow twitch
	55–65%	60–70%	Cardiovascular function Fluid balance Substrate availability		
	65–85%	70–90%	Cardiovascular function Mitochondrial density Capillary density	Aerobic	Type IIA
	85–100%	90–100%	Mitochondrial density Capillary density Lactate tolerance	Anaerobic glycolysis	
	>100%	N/A	Maximum force generation Lactate tolerance	Anaerobic glycolysis PCr	
high intensity					Fast twitch

phosphate is fully replenished and maximum effort can be repeated. This type of training produces optimum recruitment of fibres for maximum force generation.

Middle distance events rely on fast twitch fibres and on anaerobic glycolysis to sustain a high power output for 2–3 minutes. Training the muscle to use glycogen in anaerobic pathways and to clear the lactate more quickly is important. Thus middle distance runners may include high-intensity intervals of 1–3 minutes alternated with recovery periods of 1–2 minutes such that lactate builds up in the muscle but a consistently high intensity is maintained throughout the training session.

Lactic acid is always eventually reused as fuel. It can be turned back into pyruvate in the muscle cell or shunted into adjacent muscle cells and used within the mitochondria in aerobic respiration. Alternatively it is cleared into the bloodstream, converted into lactate and transported to the liver where it undergoes conversion to glucose. Fast removal of lactic acid from the muscle is reflected in quick recovery from high intensity bursts.

Longer, slower distance

Long, slow is a bit of anomaly when we look at the times of distance runners. Top-class marathon runners run each mile of the marathon faster than most of us can run one single mile. For any activity that lasts longer than a few minutes energy is supplied primarily by aerobic metabolism. The better that distance runners are at supplying and utilising oxygen within the muscles the better they are able to sustain

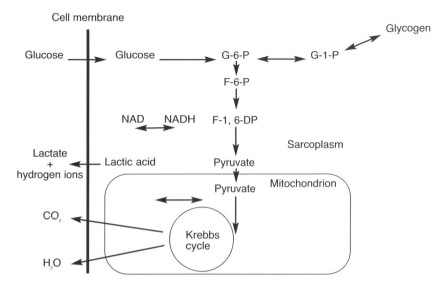

Figure 12.1 The fate of lactic acid

power over time. A combination of high MVO_2 and ability to sustain power output close to MVO_2 produces the best distance runners.

Increases in MVO_2

For the untrained there is only a small increase in stroke volume during the move from rest to exercise. For these people most of the increased cardiac output needed to facilitate the increased activity levels comes from an increase in heart rate.

While untrained individuals may increase their VO_2 max by 20 per cent with just six months training,[1] at intensities of 60–90 per cent of MVO_2, trained individuals may have reached their genetic ceiling for MVO_2 in which case they will make no further improvements to this aspect of physiology.

Maximum Exercise					
	CARDIAC OUTPUT	=	HEART RATE	×	STROKE VOLUME
UNTRAINED	22 LITRES	=	195 BPM	×	113 ml
TRAINED	35 LITRES	=	195 BPM	×	179 ml

In the trained individual, increase in stroke volume (i.e. the volume of blood ejected from the heart with each beat) increases the cardiac output dramatically. In fact, the highly trained endurance athlete has a cardiac output during maximum work equal to twice that of his sedentary counterpart.

Generally, due to their smaller body size, women have a stroke volume of about 25% less than men and correspondingly have a lower VO_2max.

In trained athletes, maximum stroke volume is reached at about 40–50 per cent of VO_2 max, so to reach peak performance for distance events the trained runner must also improve O_2 delivery to the muscles and train the metabolism such that he can sustain intensities close to VO_2max for long periods of time.

> Well-trained marathoners have been recorded training at 70–80 per cent MVO_2 for several hours. These highly trained runners can reach steady-state exercise at greater percentages of MVO_2. That is, they can work harder for longer and are more able to utilise fat at higher intensities, sparing their carbohydrate stores.

Training to increase the size and number of the mitochondria and the density of the capillary network, and to induce the type IIA muscle fibres to work aerobically has the effect of allowing the runner to maintain a higher intensity of exercise without significant lactic acid accumulation, or in other words to have a higher anaerobic threshold. Training for these changes involves training at higher intensities; 85–100 per cent of VO_2max for some of the time.

Competitive endurance events range from those taking as little as 5–6 minutes to complete to those taking several hours. Training has a different emphasis dependent on where along this continuum your sport is situated.

For high-intensity, short-duration endurance events the muscles rely primarily on glycogen as fuel. As exercise is prolonged the muscle glycogen stores are used up and there is a gradual increase in the use of fat as fuel. Those runners who are most able to utilise fat as fuel are most adapted to compete in long-duration events such as the marathon or multi-day events. For a given energy yield the oxygen demand is up to 7 per cent higher when using fat as fuel compared with using carbohydrate as fuel. As the duration of exercise increases the contribution to energy supply from fatty acids goes up and the heart rate increases to meet the muscle demands for extra oxygen.

> Moderately well-trained runners can sustain exercise with an oxygen uptake of about 50 per cent MVO_2 for about an hour. Steady state occurs after about the first five minutes of easy running, that is lactate accumulation, cardiac output and heart rate remain steady. If the running session is longer than this, heart rate and oxygen uptake progressively increase and the runner may feel fatigued. The increase in heart rate and oxygen uptake may be explained by the utilisation of fuels. Utilisation of fat requires more oxygen than utilisation of carbohydrate, thus the demand for oxygen increases with duration of exercise and there is a concomitant increase in heart rate for the same power output.[2]

The ability of the muscles to use fat as fuel is directly related to the number and size of the mitochondria. The better able the muscles are to use oxygen the better able they are to oxidise fat, thus sparing the muscle glycogen stores. One fundamental adaptation to endurance training is an increase in the number and size of the mitochondria, which occurs in both the slow twitch and the fast twitch fibres, providing that the intensity of exercise is great enough to recruit those fibres and the exercise programme is maintained for long enough (in days or weeks) to allow the adaptations to remain steady. Those muscles, or fibres within the muscle, that are not recruited do not adapt.

It takes about four or five weeks of training for the increase in mitochondrial content to reach steady state,[3] and high-intensity or long-duration sessions produce the greatest increase in mitochondrial density. Training at higher intensities recruits the fast twitch fibres. Recruiting these fibres induces an increase in mitochondria and capillary density in the type IIA fibres increasing their ability to utilise oxygen and to work aerobically. This means that anaerobic threshold is raised and a higher intensity of exercise can be sustained without building up lactic acid.

> About 50 per cent of the increase in mitochondrial density induced through training is lost after just one week of detraining and all of the adaptation is lost after 5 weeks of detraining. Furthermore, to regain the adaptations lost in one week of detraining can take up to four weeks of retraining.[4]

For races that rely on utilisation of fat as fuel training at low intensities, around 50 per cent MVO_2 for long periods of time (90 min to 2 hrs) increases the ability to mobilise and transport fat and has a psychological effect on endurance capabilities. Lactic acid accumulation interferes with the body's ability to utilise fat as fuel, thus low intensity training stresses the ability to metabolise fat. However, given that training at intensities high enough to innervate the type IIA fibres raises the anaerobic threshold and thus reduces the lactate level for any given intensity of exercise below threshold, this type of training also increases the body's ability to use fat as fuel.

> There are excellent endurance athletes who do not have startling VO_2max readings, but who can sustain intensities of 90–95 per cent VO_2max for an hour or more. Thus different training intensities are appropriate dependent on the aim of the training session and the training status of the athlete.

Type

'Type' refers to the specific training mode. For instance, the runner training on roads all the time will find running a fell race considerably more taxing as he has not prepared for this type of running. Equally a fell runner who never trains on the roads may find a road race particularly demanding because of the greater impact stress of road running and the constant, even stride that is required for road running.

Aerobic fitness

Cardiorespiratory fitness

What is the difference between cardiorespiratory fitness and aerobic fitness?

The condition of the heart, circulation and lungs together make up cardiorespiratory fitness. The heart is a muscular pump responsible for circulating blood around the body via a system of blood vessels. Arteries carry blood away from the heart, veins carry blood towards the heart and an intricate network of fine capillaries and venules link the arteries with the veins. The lungs are responsible for the exchange of gases between the body and the environment.

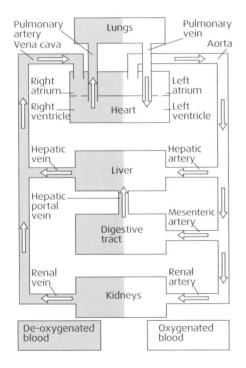

Figure 13.1 The cardiovascular system

Cardiorespiratory fitness is related to the condition of the heart, the lungs and the circulation; in other words it describes how good the body is at extracting oxygen from the air, returning carbon dioxide to the air and pumping blood around the body. Cardiovascular training (CV) is aimed at improving the efficiency of the pump, the heart. Aerobic fitness is dependent also on the condition of the working muscles and how well adapted they are to withdraw oxygen from the bloodstream and utilise it in aerobic respiration. Realistically, any improvement in cardio-vascular fitness in an untrained individual will be accompanied by improvements in the aerobic ability of the muscle; however, in highly trained individuals different types of training will target these differences and help the athlete to get the best performance.

Is a slow heart rate good for me?

There is a need for the body to regulate the speed of the pumping heart. With the onset of exercise, more oxygen is needed in the working muscles, there is more

The blood

The bloodstream carries oxygen, carbon dioxide, fuel, hormones, enzymes, heat and waste products around the body.

With the onset of exercise, more oxygen is needed in the working muscles, there is more carbon dioxide to expel from the body and excess heat must be dissipated.

carbon dioxide to expel from the body and excess heat must be dissipated so a greater flow of blood must be pumped around the body.

As we exercise, therefore, there is an increase in heart rate (HR) in an attempt to supply oxygen to meet the demand and to get rid of carbon dioxide from the working muscles. To assist the heart in this work the body also is able to regulate the internal dimensions of various blood vessels, constricting or dilating them in order to direct blood to the parts of the body where it is most needed, while maintaining blood pressure.

During rest about 5% of the blood pumped each minute is directed towards the skin. When exercising in a hot, humid environment as much as 20% is directed towards the skin in an attempt to dissipate heat. As heat loss is via perspiration we need to ensure that we drink plenty while we exercise. If we do not, we will dehydrate, affecting our blood volume, blood pressure and ability to perform.

Fluid loss can be measured by weight loss. A decrease in just 2% of your body weight equates to a decrease in performance of about 6–7%. A fluid loss of 5% of body weight equates to a decrease in performance of 30% and may result in feelings of nausea, vomiting and diarrhoea.

The heart has an internal pacemaker known as the sino-atrial node (S-A node), which spontaneously polarises and depolarises to provide stimulation for the heart to contract. This pacemaker activity is totally separate from the nervous system of the body so the heart would continue to beat at 70–80 beats per minute (BPM) under the influence of the S-A node even if all nervous fibres were cut; however, there are neural influences superimposed upon this inherent contractile rhythm.

A slow heart rate is not always a sign of fitness; some diseases are characterised by slow heart rate and some drugs artificially slow the heart rate.

Long-term exercisers exhibit changes in these neural influences and this has the effect of slowing the heart rate at rest. Therefore, healthy regular exercisers have a slower resting heart rate than healthy non-exercisers. Equally, for any given submaximal workload the heart of a trained person will beat more slowly than in the untrained state. Despite this healthy exercisers are still able to pump blood around the body effectively because, although the resting heart rate (RHR) is slower, there is more blood expelled from

A slow heart rate is not always a sign of fitness; some diseases are characterised by a slow heart rate and some drugs artificially slow the heart rate.

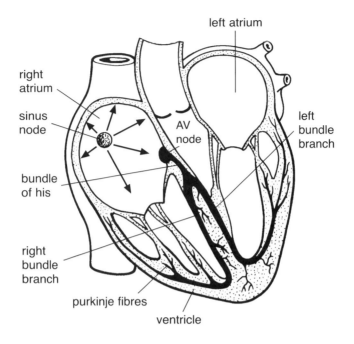

Figure 13.2 The heart's internal pacemaker

the heart with each beat; that is, they have a greater **stroke volume**. Normally a small amount of blood, about 50–70 ml, remains in the left ventricle of the heart after the heart contracts. Training enhances the force of contraction such that a greater volume of blood is ejected from the heart at each stroke. This greater stroke volume increases the **cardiac output** dramatically. In fact, during maximum work, the highly trained endurance athlete has a cardiac output equal to twice that of his sedentary counterpart.

> **Women**
> Due to their smaller body size, women generally have a stroke volume of about 25% less than that of men.

> At rest, normal **cardiac output** is about 5 litres per min. To achieve this an untrained person's heart will beat at around 70–80 BPM; however a trained person's heart will beat at around 40–50 BPM.

An increased stroke volume then, as occurs in a trained individual, causes a reduced resting heart rate as well as a significant increase in cardiac output. The increase in stroke volume may also be partly due to enhanced venous return, as the slower HR increases the time available for the heart to fill with blood. This increase in venous return during **diastole** stretches the wall of the heart (myocardium), and, in the same way that a stretched elastic band has more stored power, this causes a more powerful ejection stroke when the heart contracts.

The function of lungs is the exchange of gases between the internal environment of the body and the external environment. This gaseous exchange is achieved by utilising a muscular bellows to draw air into the lungs and force air out. Inside the lungs are tiny air sacs called alveoli, each made of a very thin

> **Stroke volume** is the amount of blood ejected from the left ventricle of the heart during contraction.
> **Cardiac output** is the volume of blood pumped out by the heart per minute and is the stroke volume × the heart rate.
> **Heart rate** × stroke volume = cardiac output.

Maximum exercise

	heart rate ×	stoke volume =	cardiac output
Untrained person	195 BPM ×	113 mls =	22 litres
Trained person	195 BPM ×	179 mls =	35 litres

semi-permeable membrane through which oxygen and carbon dioxide can pass. In the normal healthy adult there are more than 300 million of these alveoli with a total surface area that would cover half a tennis court but occupy a volume of only 4–6 litres, that is, the amount of air in a basketball.

We breathe in air from which oxygen diffuses across the walls of the alveoli into the blood capillaries. Carbon dioxide from the blood diffuses across the walls of the alveoli into the air in the lungs and is breathed out.

> **diastole**-resting phase or relaxation of cardiac muscle that allows the heart to refill with blood, and allows coronary circulation to occur.

What happens to the oxygen after it reaches the bloodstream?

The oxygen is carried in the bloodstream on the protein – haemoglobin – found in the red blood cells. When it reaches the working muscles it is given up by the haemoglobin and taken up by the muscles where it is transported to the

Effects of endurance exercise

increased stroke volume leads to

- Reduced heart rate at rest

- Reduced exercising heart rate at a given submaximal workload

- Greater cardiac output at any given heart rate

- Greater VO_2max

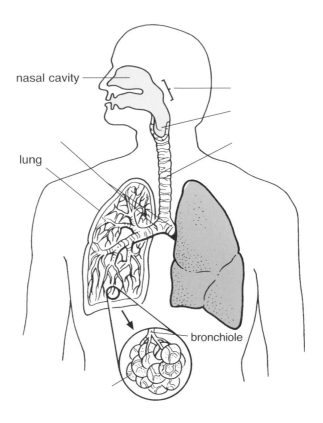

nasal cavity

lung

bronchiole

Figure 13.3 The respiratory system

Why do I feel short of breath?

We are stimulated to breathe harder, not by a lack of oxygen in the blood stream, but by an increase in carbon dioxide. In an effort to get rid of the carbon dioxide we are stimulated to breathe **out** rather than to breathe **in**.

Ventilation rate is also affected:

• when stretch receptors in lung tissue fire an automatic response;

• when there is an increase in internal body temperature;

• when there is a fall in blood pressure;

• when there is increased acidosis in the blood (as when there is a build-up of lactic acid).

When the body is at rest the most important respiratory stimulus is CO_2 pressure in the bloodstream.

mitochondria of the muscles for use in aerobic production of energy.

As we exercise, the working muscles utilise O_2 and produce CO_2, thus changing the concentration of both these gases in the blood. This changes both the **concentration gradients** and the **partial pressures** of O_2 and CO_2 in the body.

What effect does training have on the function of the lungs?

Training increases the number of capillaries surrounding the alveoli. This increased pulmonary capilliarization improves the ability of the lungs to exchange gases, that is to take oxygen into the body and get rid of carbon dioxide.

Because the diaphragm and intercostal muscles that control breathing are also trainable, regular exercise increases their ability to force air out of the lungs. Thus 'forced vital capacity', the amount of air that can be forced out of the lungs in one breath, is increased.

Concentration gradient. Gases diffuse from high concentration to low concentration along a concentration gradient.

Partial pressure is the pressure exerted by individual gases in a mixture of gases.

It is thought that in most healthy individuals the pulmonary system does not limit performance. In diseased lung, however, or if the ability to breathe is inadequate, as in people with asthma, it may be that aerobic capacity is limited by a failure of breathing to keep pace with the body's demand for oxygen.

The muscles that cause us to breathe, the diaphragm and intercostal muscles, themselves utilise oxygen to provide the energy for contraction. In people with severely diseased lungs, the oxygen cost of breathing may reach as much as 40% of the total oxygen cost of exercising.

What effect does exercise have on the exchange of gases?

After only four weeks of training the amount of oxygen extracted from the air and utilised by the body is increased, independently of the amount of air being moved in and out of the lungs. Thus we don't have to breathe so hard to extract the same amount of oxygen from the air. This means that a smaller amount of air is breathed at any given submaximal workload, therefore the energy cost of breathing is reduced.

Maximum aerobic capacity (VO_2max)

Maximum aerobic capacity (VO_2max), or aerobic power, is the maximum amount of oxygen that you can extract from the air and utilise in the working muscles for the aerobic production of energy. In other words, the amount of oxygen you can use when exercising at very high intensities. VO_2max is affected by body size, gender, and age and is measured in litres/min and often expressed relative to body weight, in ml per kilo of body weight per minute.

The average man has a VO_2max of 45ml/L/min, whereas, on average, world-class cross-country skiers have a VO_2max of around 86.7ml/L/min.

VO_2max is trainable but has a genetic ceiling; that is, one is born with a set limit on VO_2max. Very high values have been recorded in elite endurance athletes. The higher the VO_2max the more able that person is to utilise oxygen to fuel exercise, therefore the greater the potential for high-level performance in endurance sports.

Average VO_2max levels for women are about 65–70% of that of men. The mean value for a 65-year-old man is the same as that of a 25-year-old woman.[1]

Training can enhance VO_2max but only within a person's genetic ceiling. In other words, training can only help you to make best use of the potential with which you were born.

⑭ Muscle

Muscle fibres

Muscles are made up of fibres and within every muscle there are different fibre types. These fibre types differ in contractile speed, in enzyme characteristics and in **metabolic enzyme profile**. Muscle is therefore classified into different fibre types. Muscle fibres have been characterised as slow twitch and fast twitch fibres, based on the time it takes for them to reach peak tension once they are stimulated to contract. Slow twitch fibres are also called type I fibres, while fast twitch fibres are called type II fibres.

> **Metabolic enzyme profile.** Muscle fibres can be differentiated by distinguishing the enzymes characteristic of the different energy systems that they use.

However, muscle fibres can also be classified based on their metabolic properties, so that type I fibres might be termed 'slow oxidative' fibres. They have a lot of mitochondria and oxidative enzymes and a plentiful supply of capillaries and so are well adapted for aerobic respiration. Type II fibres may be termed 'fast glycolytic' fibres. They are well adapted for anaerobic respiration, and they reach peak tension very quickly.

Are there more than two fibre types?

Based on metabolic properties type II or fast twitch muscle fibres can be further divided into subcategories. At least two types of fast twitch fibre have been identified. Type IIB fibres are known as 'fast glycolytic' (FG) and type IIA fibres as 'fast oxidative glycolytic' (FOG). The FG fibres store lots of **glycogen** and have high levels of the enzymes necessary for producing energy

> **Glycogen** is the body's store of carbohydrate.
>
> **Oxidative enzymes** are the enzymes involved in aerobic metabolism.

anaerobically (without oxygen) but they contain relatively few mitochondria. The FOG fibres are similar to these FG fibres, but are capable of adapting and increasing their ability to utilise oxygen, by increasing their number of mitochondria, **oxidative enzymes** and blood capillaries.

These adaptations occur with training and result in a person being able to work at higher intensities while utilising aerobic respiration; in other words, with more endurance at higher intensities.

Slow twitch fibres are fatigue-resistant and so are associated with endurance events.

Strength

Absolute strength requires high total force production irrespective of the rate of force production, and is a function of the number of fibre types, both slow and fast, that are recruited and the size of the muscle.

The strength of a muscle is directly proportional to the cross-sectional area of the muscle. Thus a weak elephant will still be stronger than a strong horse simply because its muscles are bigger. For this reason in strength sports such as powerlifting it would be unfair for a large person to compete against a small person; thus strength-related sports are split into weight classes for competition.

Do I use fast twitch or slow twitch fibres when I train for strength?

In order to perform one maximal lift as in powerlifting, all the available muscle fibres must be recruited, both slow and fast twitch. The type IIB fibres will fatigue during that one maximal effort and so that lift will not be achieved again until recovery of those type II fibres is complete. However, the powerlifter would immediately be able to lift a lighter weight that recruited type I fibres and very probably, with this lighter weight, would achieve more than one repetition.

Increases in strength are partly due to neurogenic changes; that is, changes in the nervous system, and partly due to changes in the contractile elements of the muscle – the myofilaments.

Initially, improvements in strength come from learning to recruit more fibres to achieve the task, or, more accurately, learning to recruit as many fibres as possible in the right sequence to achieve the task with greater efficiency and force production. Further increases in strength occur at a myogenic level. The myofilaments actin and myosin found within the muscle increase in size and number, so increasing their contractile force.

So to get stronger do I need to get bigger?

Many athletes are concerned that if they put on weight they will have more weight to carry around and will therefore become slower, so they shy away from strength training. In reality great strength gains can be made without any increase in weight at all. By working at very specific strength training, increases in strength due to neurogenic changes may benefit the athlete. For instance, a shot putter may put a heavier shot in training than in competition. A swimmer may use hand paddles to increase the resistance afforded by the water. A cross-country skier may spend a lot of time double-poling uphill to increase upper body strength.

Further strength gains may be due to changes in the size of the muscle; however, this is not necessarily counterproductive.

Increases in muscle mass, especially in older athletes, are often accompanied by reduction in fat mass.[1] As muscle is metabolically active this has the effect of increasing the metabolic rate and helping to maintain low body fat levels.[2] Often athletes starting a strength training programme notice that when they stand on the scales their weight hasn't changed despite the improved muscle tone. The increase in muscle has been accompanied by a reduction in body fat and so overall weight has not been affected. Further, whereas fat is in effect dead weight for the athlete to carry around, muscle produces force. Often a slight increase in weight is offset by the much greater increase in power.

Finally, athletic activity produces large forces in the joints. It is the musculature around the joint that counteracts these forces, stabilising it and holding it together during sport. Many injuries occur and reoccur because the **fixator muscles** around the joint are not strong enough to do this job, thus strengthening these muscles may prevent injury and allow the athlete to train more consistently and improve performance.

> **Fixator muscles** check unwanted movement in a joint or joint complex.

Strength and health

Many of our everyday activities involve strength: carrying shopping and moving furniture, for instance. Lower-back pain is often a result of poor lifting technique in everyday situations. The erector spinae muscles of the back need to be capable of applying enough force to offset the considerable load acting in an anterior direction on the facet joints and on the intervertebral discs during lifting. They need to be capable of holding the spine erect against the weight of a load pulling the body forwards.

> **Vertebrae** are the individual bones that make up the spine.
>
> **Hyperextension** refers to over-extension of a joint.

Not only do the back muscles need to be strong when lifting but also the abdominal muscles need to be strong enough to fixate the **vertebrae** and to prevent **hyperextension** of the spine when carrying loads.

The National Fitness Survey (1992)[3] reported very poor leg power in the UK, reflecting the trend in much of the Western world. Without enough strength in the legs and trunk to enable you to bend down and lift correctly (with a straight back and bent knees) you risk damaging your back every time you pick up so much as a pencil or piece of paper from the floor. Position statements from the US Surgeon General's Office, based on worldwide research upholds strength training as the key factor in maintaining functional ability, health and independence as we age.[4]

Doesn't increase in strength cause reduced flexibility?

A quick look at the range of movement (ROM) evident in Olympic weightlifters belies the myth that strength training reduces flexibility. As with most exercise, much is dependent on how it is carried out. If a full range of movement is used during strength work then a full range will be maintained. Further, as functional flexibility is reliant not only on **passive range of movement** but also on **active range** then strengthening exercises may be found to improve flexibility and counteract the potential for injury to the muscles and joints. In a study on physical education students it was found that strengthening exercises did not significantly reduce the passive flexibility scores but were found to stabilise the joints by increasing the active ROM, thus reducing the difference between the active and passive ranges.[5]

> **Passive range of movement** is demonstrated when joint movement is assisted by an outside force.
>
> **Active range of movement** is the range of movement when only the muscles affecting that movement are used.

Power

Power is the product of both force and the rate at which that force can be applied.

> Power = speed × strength

Power combines the speed and the force of contraction, with peak output generally occurring at around 30 per cent of maximum velocity (figure 15.2). Dependent on an individual's power-generating capacity, application of peak power in the quadriceps can allow for that person to just manage to rise from their chair or cause the person to leap into the air!

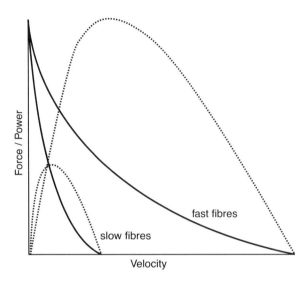

For power athletes such as sprinters, throwers, jumpers, and Olympic weightlifters a large number of fast twitch fibres capable of generating peak power quickly is therefore advantageous.

Multiple sprints sports are characterised by an ability to keep repeating maximal sprint efforts with short recovery periods. The ability to recover quickly from and reproduce maximal efforts is more important in these sports than maximal achievable power. Nevertheless many world-class team players would also make world class sprinters.

Figure 14.2 Force-velocity relationship of skeletal muscle in slow, and fast fibres. Power-velocity relationships are shown in broken lines. Source: Medicine and Sport Science
editors: M Hebbelinck, Brussels; R.J. Shepphard, Toronto, Ont.

Endurance

Endurance is dependent on repeated submaximal-intensity contractions. However, both type I and type IIA fibres are responsible for prolonged exercise of submaximal intensity, thus speed in endurance events requires that we train the type IIA fibres to be more able to utilise oxygen and so accumulate less lactate. Therefore endurance cannot be considered only in terms of fibre type recruitment but must also be considered in metabolic terms.

Fatigue in endurance activity is partly a function of build-up of lactate and partly due to draining the muscle glycogen stores. Repleting the muscle glycogen stores may take as long as two days.

Endurance training increases the size and number of the mitochondria in both type I and type IIA muscle fibres, thus increasing the aerobic ability of the muscle and the ability to utilise fat as fuel, which is related to the size and number of the mitochondria. This in turn spares muscle glycogen stores during prolonged low-intensity exercise, and also reduces lactate production, thus prolonging the time to fatigue and facilitating higher-intensity exercise without fatigue.[6]

Can muscle fibre type be changed with training?

Each muscle or group of muscles has an associated nerve fibre that innervates the muscle to contract, and it is this nerve fibre that directs muscle fibre type. Only changing the nerve will change the fibre type. There is no conclusive evidence that it is possible to convert slow twitch fibres to fast twitch fibres, or fast twitch fibres to slow twitch through training. Although sprinters show large proportions of fast twitch fibres and elite endurance athletes have large proportions of slow twitch fibres it is unclear whether this is a result of training or whether genetics has played a role in the selection of their sport.

Endurance training at high intensities recruits the type I and type IIA fibres and loads them repeatedly with little or no rest. The body responds by developing more mitochondria and aerobic enzymes and increasing the surrounding capillary network. High-intensity endurance training therefore trains the type IIA fibres to utilise oxygen in the aerobic production of energy. Whereas this does nothing to enhance their maximum power output, it does increase sustainable power, allowing a higher intensity of exercise to be fuelled by aerobic respiration and reducing the build-up of lactic acid.

Biopsies of elite endurance athletes show that they have almost no IIB fibres, but have a significant percentage of IIA fibres. Whether these athletes are born with a very high percentage of type IIA fibres and so are able to become elite endurance athletes, or whether endurance training over many years causes the type IIB fibres to transmute into type IIA fibres is unclear.

> In **needle biopsies** a needle with a canula is inserted into the muscle tissue and a small piece of muscle tissue is withdrawn.

Can I train to be a better sprinter?

Training for sprint and power sports loads all the fast twitch fibres type IIA and IIB for power. During maximal-intensity exercise of 5–6 seconds duration, by use of the

> During brief maximal exercise of 5–6 seconds duration, power outputs 2–3 times that at VO_2max can be achieved.
>
> - Muscle lactate increases by around 200%
> - Creatine phosphate contributes about 50% of ATP resynthesis
> - Glycolysis contributes about 50% of ATP resynthesis

> It is suggested that sprint training can increase creatine phosphate and also that it may be possible to do the same by supplementing the diet with creatine.[7]

creatine phosphate system and the stored adenosine tri-phosphate power, output at 2–3 times higher than at VO_2max can be tolerated.[8] It is suggested that sprint training increases the muscle use of creatine phosphate and the enzymes associated with anaerobic metabolism, so that the type IIA fibres become well adapted for speed but not so well adapted for endurance.[9]

The muscle fibre does not distinguish between the force needed to lift a weight and the force needed to sprint or jump. It simply is innervated to contract and supply force, thus recruitment of fibres in sprint training may lead to greater muscle mass, which in turn may lead to greater power output and less fatigue during any given high power output.

Are strength training and endurance training compatible?

The answer to this question is: 'That depends.' It depends on:

- what type of strength and endurance training you are doing;

- how well trained you already are;

- what your exercise mode is; and

- what you hope will be the outcome.

> Studies that use improved performance as their measure often conclude that improved strength is of benefit to the endurance athlete. This improvement in performance may be a function of greater sustainable power output, of improved mechanical efficiency or of fewer injuries.

A large amount of scientific research has studied strength training alongside running and the results have been equivocal.[10] The difficulty for researchers is that performance is multifaceted rather than dependent on a single component, and that different people respond in different ways dependent on their genetics, age, gender and training status.

So is strength training good for the endurance athlete?

Any increase in muscle mass without a proportional increase in muscle oxidative capacity might actually be viewed as detrimental to the performance of the endurance athlete, so research that measures VO_2max, mitochondrial density or the enzyme profile of the fibre types, draws the conclusion that strength training is detrimental to endurance, especially in activities such as running and cross-country skiing where the body weight must be supported.[11]

However, studies that use improved performance as their measure often conclude that improved strength is of benefit to the endurance athlete. This improvement in performance may be a function of greater sustainable power output, of improved mechanical efficiency or of fewer injuries. It would seem sensible that endurance athletes such as cross-country skiers, rowers and paddlers who rely on either upper body muscle or a combination of upper and lower body muscle would benefit from greater upper body strength. Certainly wheelchair marathoners rely on good upper body muscle mass and strength.

Is endurance training good for the strength athlete?

If increased strength is the aim of the athlete, endurance training of relatively short duration, such that it does not deplete glycogen stores, would seem to have no detrimental effect; however, long-duration training that thoroughly depletes the glycogen stores forces the body to utilise protein and break down muscle as an energy source and is therefore **catabolic** in nature. This type of training may limit strength gains.

> **Catabolism** is the breaking down of muscle tissue – the destructive phase of metabolism.
>
> **Anabolism** is the building up of muscle tissue – the constructive phase of metabolism.

The strength–endurance continuum

Strength and endurance are not two separate issues but rather constitute a continuum. At the one end of the continuum we have absolute strength requiring maximum muscular force to be generated in one singular voluntary contraction. That is a force that will overcome a resistance once, but only once. In weight training terms it is the ability to lift a weight once only (1RM).

> **1RM** – one repetition maximum, the resistance needed to limit the lifter to one repetition only. A second repetition of the exercise cannot be achieved.

At the other end of the continuum is the ability to apply a muscular force repeatedly. This could be any number of contractions and in endurance activities may be many hundreds of contractions repeated. In strength training terms this end of the continuum would be represented by any number above 15 contractions (usually between 15RM and 25RM).

Strength solidus endurance crossover

If a muscle or group of muscles is extremely weak, such as after prolonged bed rest, then any activity, even if normally classified as an endurance activity, is likely to increase the strength capabilities of that group of muscles.

Similarly, as each motor unit becomes stronger, as happens with heavy resistance training, then fewer motor units are needed to complete a given maximum workload, thus creating a greater motor unit reserve and increasing endurance capabilities.

The changes in a muscle are specific to the stimulus placed upon it. If the stimulus is of low intensity and towards the endurance end of the continuum then the changes will be to the slow twitch muscle and will improve its endurance capabilities.

If the stimulus is of very high intensity then the changes will involve the fast twitch muscle and will improve its strength capabilities.

'The perfect way is only difficult for those who pick and choose. Do not like, do not dislike; all will then be clear.'

Bruce Lee

Is multi-sport training the only sensible way to train?

Is multi-sport training the only sensible way to train? As always with fitness the answer has to be: 'That depends'. However, one thing is certain and that is that while an unstructured programme may provide you with increases in fitness or performance levels, to be as successful as possible, a multi-sport training programme has to be structured.

A haphazard approach to multi-sport training will at best give haphazard results and at worst will increase the risk of injury. Understanding the principles of multi-sport training will assist you greatly in designing training programmes that maximise benefits while minimising risks.

Programme structure

There are many ways to write a training programme. However, a paramount principle is that a structured approach will give the best results.

It is estimated that without a structured programme an athlete will reach only 75% of his or her potential. A haphazard approach may predispose an athlete to injury by overtraining, by overdeveloping some muscles and underdeveloping others or inadequately preparing for the physiological stress of competition.

'Genotype is also strongly involved in determining the response to regular exercise and to an increase in fitness.'

Claude Bouchard[1]

Each person is a unique individual and each of us responds to training in a different way, thus we each need our own individual training programme. Utilising someone else's programme may provide us with guidelines but will fail to take into account each individual's particular circumstances, unique history, unique genetic ability and response to training.

Playing God

If we were to play God to a world, we would first look at the whole to decide what we wanted for the future of that world. Then we would need to examine each nation and ensure that, without adversely affecting the nations around it or with whom it interacted, it was progressing in a way that would enhance its future and that of the world. However, rather than get bogged down in the progression of one nation only, every so often we would need to take a general overview so as to make sure that we were still moving into the future that we had envisaged.

To write a multi-sport training programme we play God to the body. We must look at the whole multifaceted picture and determine exactly what we want from this programme. Then we must examine all the individual pieces and make sure that each individual piece is set up right. Periodically we must stand back from the whole picture and make sure that it still all fits together well.

Programming for health/fitness

When putting a multi-sport training programme together for general health and fitness purposes, rather than for any specific competitive achievement, the immediate issue is to decide which activities you like to do. Essentially a mix of activities that includes strength, endurance and flexibility for both upper and lower body will give an all-round fitness base. When picking training modes you should look at a balance of these three areas of fitness. For instance, swimming provides endurance and flexibility, so adding in a strength-based activity such as a strength circuit will provide the balance. T'ai chi provides flexibility and strength, so adding a cardiovascular activity such as walking will provide balance. Having decided on the training modes, then training frequency, intensity and time can be manipulated to ensure a safe and effective programme.

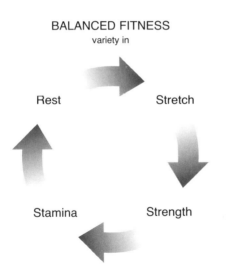

BALANCED FITNESS
variety in

Rest   Stretch

Stamina   Strength

Figure 15.1 All-round fitness

How often, how hard, how much, for health?

The ACSM guidelines suggest that for health, aerobic exercise of a moderate intensity should be undertaken for 30 minutes on most days of the week. For fitness, aerobic exercise of a vigorous intensity should be undertaken for 20 minutes three times a week, and two strength training sessions each incorporating 8–10 repetitions and 1–2 sets of 8–10 exercises covering most of the body should be achieved.

How this is done in a training programme for health then depends on the circumstances, likes and dislikes of the individual:

- How often can you realistically make time to train?

- For how long can you train at each session?

- What do you like to do?

Examples:

1. John works a regular week and spends time with his family at weekends. He knows that every evening he can spend a total of one hour and 35 minutes training. This allows him 20 minutes travelling time from work to the gym, 30 minutes training time, 15 minutes showering time and 30 minutes travelling time from the gym to home. He then arrives home at around 7.30 p.m. For his family find this quite tolerable. Training at the weekend would change this – weekends are strictly family time. John likes to train with weights and on cardiovascular machines, except steppers, and he also likes to cycle.

He sets up his training programme to allow him three gym-based sessions of 30 minutes and 2 cycle sessions. On Tuesdays and Thursdays he goes straight home from work and then goes out cycling from home. This allows him an extra 20 minutes as he has cut out travelling to the gym. So on these days he cycles for 50 minutes to an hour. On Mondays, Wednesdays and Fridays he goes home via the gym. Mondays and Wednesdays he does a strength-based circuit on resistance machines. On Fridays he joins in a circuit class that mixes aerobic work and strength/endurance work. The class lasts an hour, so if he and his wife have anything planned on a Friday he may miss the class.

Table 15.1 John's fitness programme

	Activity	Duration
Monday	Strength-based resistance machines plus flexibility	30 min
Tuesday	Cycle plus flexibility	50–60 min
Wednesday	Strength-based resistance machines plus flexibility	30 min
Thursday	Cycle plus flexibility	50–60 min
Friday	Circuit class aerobic and muscular endurance	60 min

So most weeks John follows the ACSM guidelines and does a total of three aerobic sessions of at least 20 minutes in length and achieves two strength-based sessions. His stretching exercises are done on the floor at home in the evenings.

Table 15.2 Frances's fitness programme

	Activity	Duration
Monday	Run	30 min
Tuesday	Walk	30 min
Wednesday	Dance; muscular endurance and flexibility	90 min
Thursday	Walk	30 min
Friday	Circuit class aerobic and muscular strength endurance	60 min
Saturday	Run	30 min
Sunday	Water circuit; strength and endurance	60 min

2. Frances is at college. Her timetable allows that some days she has a free afternoon or morning. She works three evenings a week in a restaurant and has varying degrees of studying to complete in her own time. For her, scheduling regular day-by-day activity is, to say the least, difficult. She cannot afford to join a gym, and in any case dislikes training in fitness studios or gyms.

Frances sets up her programme by attending one dance class on Wednesday afternoons. As she is studying drama this fits in nicely with her studies, and also achieves one session of mixed activity with flexibility worked in. It is difficult to categorise this session as it is sometimes aerobic and sometimes anaerobic, so she counts it as muscular endurance and flexibility.

Two days a week Frances runs for 30 minutes. Every day of the week she walks to and from college. This involves 15 minutes brisk walking, adding up to half an hour every day. On Sunday of most weeks she attends a water circuit class, which involves a mix of strength and endurance work.

Frances, through dance and circuit training, running and walking, also meets the ACSM minimum guidelines for health and is most of the way to achieving their minimum guidelines for fitness.

The body adapts only to unaccustomed stress

For both John and Frances, once the body has adapted to this training so that it is no longer difficult, they will plateau at that fitness level. The body adapts only to unaccustomed stress. If they have no wish to improve further that is fine. They are meeting the guidelines for fitness and health. However if they want to improve further in any aspect they will have to change something. They can change frequency, intensity time or type of exercise in order to alter their programme and initiate further improvements. Without a goal it is difficult to decide what to change. It maybe that change is forced upon them. May be a new instructor starts to take the class and alters the intensity of the training or the length of the class. Maybe Frances moves further from college and now has to walk for 25 minutes each way, changing the duration of her training sessions. Maybe John buys a mountain bike and starts to ride off-road as well as on-road, automatically adding more upper body work to his programme.

John now, however, is pleased with his improvements in fitness and decides to enter a 100-mile sponsored bike ride to raise money for a local charity. He now has a specific achievement goal. He has become a sportsperson, and will have to plan his programme more specifically if he is to be successful .

Structured programme building for a challenge event or competition

If the multi-sport training programme is leading to a challenge, event or competition then the programming has to be more focused and a more scientific approach is valuable.

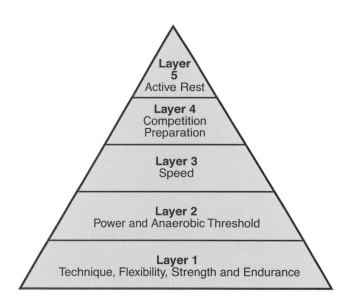

Training pyramid

Many aspects of fitness training need a firm base from which to build. For instance, power is a combination of strength and speed, but power training subjects the body to extreme forces and must therefore be done from a firm foundation of strength, both to facilitate the power and to protect the

Figure 15.2 Training pyramid

musculo-skeletal system from injury.

The first priority then in building a training programme is a firm base on top of which refinements such as speed, power and reaction time may be added. Finally event or competition preparation may include tapering, psychological preparation, nutritional preparation etc.

Periodisation

Training then can be systematically split up into training phases or layers. Whereas there may be considerable overlap of one phase into another, splitting it up in this way allows the athlete to focus mainly on one or two limiting factors during phases of training, thus maximising the efficiency of her or his time. The whole training programme that leads up to an event is often called a macrocycle, that is, a cycle of training that incorporates everything. The big picture!

Breaking down the training period or macrocycle into phases allows for focusing on the weak link. These phases are often called mesocycles.

A break from tradition

Traditionally competitive sports split the training macrocycle into four mesocycles.

- Conditioning

- Preparation

- Competition

- Recovery

02-Feb			Macrocycle			27-Jul	
February	March		April	May	June	July	
2 9 16 23	2 9 16 23 30		6 13 20 27	4 11 18 25	1 8 15 22 29	6 13 20 27	

	Mesocycles		
02-Feb	06-Apr	01-Jun	06-Jul
conditioning	preparation	competition	recovery

Figure 15.3 A macrocycle/mesocycle programme

In reality how many mesocycles are included is less relevant than the concept of this system and the end result for the individual. Thus the structure that I have laid out below breaks from tradition and splits the macrocycle into five phases. I have included two conditioning phases as mesocycle 1 and mesocycle 2. This allows for separate training aims, such as strength and power, to be delineated.

Mesocycle 1

The first mesocycle occurs out of season and is used to ensure adequate skill, flexibility, endurance and strength to support the rest of the training and competition. This mesocycle should be used to focus on technique, to improve flexibility, to build endurance, to rehabilitate from any injury and to correct muscular imbalances that may predispose towards injury. Thus for a marathon runner this mesocycle may include a considerable amount of lower body flexibility and strength work, while for a canoeist the emphasis will be on upper body work and on technique. For sports involving power, where increased muscle mass may be of benefit, muscle hypertrophy utilising high-volume high-intensity weight training may come into this mesocycle.

One of my clients whose sport was hang-gliding and who was naturally of light build spent this mesocycle building muscle so that he had the weight to control his glider.

Multi-sport training is an ideal tool to use in mesocycle 1. Improvements to central circulation are training-specific rather than sport-specific, so changes to the heart and central circulation occur whether we run or cycle, for instance. Likewise multi-sport training using weight training, circuit training or other forms of resistive work may be used to increase strength.

> Multi-sport training is an ideal tool to use in Mesocycle 1.
>
> T'ai chi may be used to increase strength and balance for rock-climbing. Ballet dancing may be used to improve flexibility, grace and presentation skills for posing in bodybuilding.

Mesocycle 2

Mesocycle 2 is used to build on endurance or power. Thus the endurance athlete would increase mileage to ensure the ability to cope with the racing mileage. For instance, a marathon runner would build up to just below marathon distance while a 10-kilometre runner might build up to a great distance, so that running 10 kilometres feels easy.

During this mesocycle an ice-hockey player might concentrate on increased power and, towards the end of this mesocycle and the beginning of the next, on being able to recover from and repeat that power output.

In sports where power output is important, plyometric training, jumping, bounding and leaping may be included. Mesocycle 1 should become more specifically related to the sport; however, multi-sport training may still prove useful. For instance, a distance runner who was previously plagued by injuries when embarking on high-mileage training may still include a fair amount of cycling or in-line skating. This would enable him or her to increase the volume of endurance training without greatly increasing the amount of impact on the joints. Equally this athlete may continue with strength training, though at a reduced volume, in order to minimise muscular imbalance and maintain muscle strength, thus stabilising joints that were previously prone to injury. Flexibility work in the form of dance or martial arts may also be continued.

The power athlete might now reduce the volume of strength training, utilising lower repetition and sets but higher load and increased speed of movement, and should shift towards more sport-specific and multijoint exercises such as bench press, deadlift and lunges.

Mesocycle 3

Mesocycle 3 is where speed, agility and reaction time are built into the programme. Also during this mesocycle skill work and – for team sports – drills are practised. The

01-Dec			Macrocycle				27-Jul	
Dec	Jan	Feb	Mar	Apr	May	Jun	Jul	
1 8 15 22 29	5 12 19 26	2 9 16 23	2 9 16 23 30	6 13 20 27	4 11 18 25	1 8 15 22 29	6 13 20 27	

Mesocycles			
01-Dec	16-Feb	08-Jun	20-Jul
phase one	phase two	phase three	Taper
Strength, flexibility, address muscle imbalances, endurance, technique	build up endurance more specific strength	speed	race prepar
Weight Training for increased strength-utilise isolation exercise to target strength for joint stability	running; increase distance add in hill work, threshold work and intervals. cycling	low volume training specific to joint stability. Running simulating	nutrition and psycho prepar
Tai Chi running cycling, swimming	T'ai chi and/or flexibility work weight training sports-specific multijoint exercises	race conditions: interval and threshold work	

Figure 15.4 Example: endurance athlete's phased programme utilising multi-sport training

endurance athlete will build up to work at race pace and conditions and may compete in time trials and minor races. Fell runners and mountain marathoners would spend much training time on the hills during this mesocycle, if possible on terrain similar to that on which they will race. Mountain bikers similarly will attempt to simulate race conditions. Multiple-sprint athletes will work on speed, repeatable power and bursts of speed, agility reaction time and skill. Where matches are part of

01-Dec			Macrocycle				31-Aug	
Dec	Jan	Feb	Mar	Apr	May	Jun	Jul	Aug
1 8 15 22 29	5 12 19 26	2 9 16 23	2 9 16 23 30	6 13 20 27	4 11 18 25	1 8 15 22 29	6 13 20 27	3 10 17 24 31

Mesocycles			
01-Dec	16-Mar	01-Jun	27-Jul
phase one	phase two	phase three	taper
Strength and endurance flexibility, skill. running, cycling, indoor rowing weight training, circuit training flexibility, skill drills	power, anaerobic endurance psychological preparation running and indoor rowing; build in interval training, flexibility plyometric circuits weight training - using multiple joint and power lifts such as power clean	anaerobic recovery, speed, agility reaction sport specific skill drills, reaction time and agility, strength trainingon specific to joint stability, psychological preparation	skill and speed. nutritional and low volume training concentrating on skill and speed psychological preparation

Figure 15.5 Example: multiple-sprint athlete's phased programme utilising multi-sport training

extended tournaments these conditions should also be simulated.

Strength athletes such as powerlifters would become very sport-specific in this mesocycle, decreasing the volume and increasing the intensity of work, simulating competition by attempting one-repetition maximum lifts. During this mesocycle bodybuilders would be reducing fat levels and practising posing routines. Where possible training time should match the time of day of the competition.

For single-sport athletes multi-sport training should be much reduced in this mesocycle, as at this time when training volume is decreasing and training intensity is increasing, sport-specific training is vital to achieving the best performance.

Mesocycle 4

Mesocycle 4 is taper for the event. The length of the taper is dependent on the length of the event. A long taper is required for distance athletes, a shorter taper for sprint athletes. During the taper there is a decrease in volume of training while intensity is kept high. Accompanying this may be a change to psychological and nutritional preparation.

Where there is a competitive season this mesocycle may include the main part of it where the aim is to maintain or improve performance levels.

Mesocycle 5

Mesocycle 5 is a rest mesocycle, consisting of active rest for 1–4 weeks before the whole process starts again in preparation for the next season. Cross training is very appropriate to this mesocycle, training being low volume, low intensity and low pressure/stress.

Microcycles

Once the mesocycles are set up, each one progressing a particular part of the training, then each week's training can be planned.

The mesocycles can be split up into smaller sections. These are called microcycles and are very often each one week long, although they don't have to be. Now the training level can be progressed from one microcycle to the next planning how many

Mescocycles				
04-Aug	3-Nov	16-Feb	25-May	31-Aug
kayak	base 1	base 2	speed	competition

Microcycles				
04-Aug (13 weeks)		kayak		
team to kayak		skill training – kayak strength and endurance aimed specifically at kayak navigation improve body composition		
4-Aug	11 Aug	18-Aug	25-Aug	01-Sep
7 days	7 days	7 days	7 days	7 days
cycle 1	cycle 1	cycle 2	cycle 2	cycle 2
run x 3	run x 3	run x 3	run x 4	run x 4
weights x 2	weights x 3	weights x 3	weights x 3	weights x 3
kayak x 1	kayak x 1	kayak x 1	kayak x 1	kayak x 1
row x 3	row x 3	row x 3	row x 3	row x 3

Figure 15.6 Mesocycles divided into microcycles

Current cycle 1 run x 3 weights x 2 kayak x 1 row x 3
Microcycle
Details:

Date	Type of Exercise	Intensity	Time/Dur	Notes
10-Aug Sun				
11-Aug Mon				
12-Aug Tue	run/row			1 hour very easy-easy row 20 min
13-Aug Wed	weights			5 sets to failure upper body
14-Aug Thu	kayak			2 hours steady
15-Aug Fri	run			1.5 hours run
17-Aug Sun				
18-Aug Mon	run/row			30 mins, row 3,500 17.12.4
19-Aug Tue	weights			5 sets to failure
20-Aug Wed	cycle/swim			
21-Aug Thu	kayak			
22-Aug Fri				
23-Aug Sat				
24-Aug Sun	run			9 miles ish-hilly
25-Aug Mon				
26-Aug Tue	run/row			45 mins run; 1/1 min inte ints x 5 x 2 row
27-Aug Wed	weights/run			5 sets to failure

Figure 15.7 Microcycle daily programme

sessions of each discipline and the nature of that session.

The mesocycles are split up into microcycles and the training level can be progressed from one microcycle to the next planning how many sessions of each discipline

Daily plans
Once each microcycle or each week of training is planned the training can be planned on a daily basis.

Individual sessions
Finally individual sessions can be planned on each day.

Why do some athletes change their training at different times of the year?
As you can see from the training mesocycles it is possible to alter the training focus at different times of the year in order to achieve improved performance. Many individuals simply add in extra work, always supposing that more is better. This is not the case. In fact, to benefit from increased intensity in training it is often necessary to reduce the total training volume. Increasing the intensity increases the stress on the body thus necessitating longer recovery time.

Reducing training volume can be done by reducing either frequency or time or a combination of both. Thus volume of training will also change, and at different times of the year when the individual is in different periods or mesocycles of training, both the volume and intensity will change.

Session Plan Design					
Session Details: 11-Sep Mon		weights	10 reps	6 sets	
Description:					
Exercise	wt	wt	wt	wt	wt
bench press					
incline press					
cable crossover					
chins widegrip					
lat pulldown to chest					
straight arm pulldown					
bench row					
shoulder press					
lateral raise					

Coaching Instructions: Use 10 rm for all exercises
continue with same plan but incease to 6 sets from September

Figure 15.8 Individual session programme

Training Load

Overall training load is often used as a measurement and can be manipulated in such a way that when volume of training is high intensity is low and vice versa.

Training load is often measured by somehow combining intensity and volume. For instance, a runner may measure intensity by perceived exertion measured between 1 and 5 and volume by time in minutes. In one week she or he might run five days in total, which include one long slow run, two runs at a steady pace, one threshold run and one interval session of 5 × 3 minute intervals (see table 15.3).

The next week she or he may run six days in total, including one long slow run, three runs at a steady pace, one threshold run and one interval session of 6 × 3 minute intervals (see table 15.4). The total training load has increased by 132 from week 1 to week 2. In this instance the training load is not a specific measure but simply gives an estimation of by how much the training load is increasing or decreasing. If in week 2 the two steady runs became a swim and a run and the long

Table 15.3 Five-day training load

Day	Time (mins)	Reps	Total time	Intensity	Load	Load, running total
Mon	40	1	40	2	80	80
Tues	3	5	15	4	60	140
Thurs	60	1	60	2	120	260
Fri	90	1	90	1	90	350
Sun	20	1	20	3	60	410
					Total load	**410**

run became a cycle but the intensity and time remained the same, then the total training load would be the same (see table 15.5). Of course, the physiological stress may be less as the multi-sport training would take away some of the repetition and joint impact problems that can occur with single sport training such as running.

Table 15.4 Six-day training load

Day	Time (mins)	Reps	Total time	Intensity	Load	Load, running total
Mon	40	1	40	2	80	80
Tues	3	6	18	4	72	152
Thurs	60	1	60	2	120	272
Fri	90	1	90	1	90	362
Sat	60	1	60	2	120	482
Sun	20	1	20	3	60	542
					Total load	542

By watching the training load it is possible to make sure that the programming is progressing at a reasonable rate, with no sudden large jumps in volume or intensity, and also that easier recovery weeks and tapers are built into the programme.

For weight training the training load may use repetitions and sets to calculate load. Or it may be more sophisticated and utilise total repetitions and resistance, in which case it would have to be calculated per lift and then added together (see table 15.7).

As you see, the more complex the system the more accurate the tracking of load becomes; however, a simple tracking of load estimation may be just enough to ensure that the training is progressing in the right direction, that it is either

Table 15.5 Six-day training load with activities varied

Day	Mode and time in mins		Reps	Total time	Intensity	Load	Load, running total
Mon	run	40	1	40	2	80	80
Tues	run	3	6	18	4	72	152
Thurs	swim	60	1	60	2	120	272
Fri	cycle	90	1	90	1	90	362
Sat	run	60	1	60	2	120	482
Sun	run	20	1	20	3	60	542
						Total load	542

Table 15.6 Weight training load

Day	Mode	Reps	Sets	Load	Load, running total
Mon	weights	10	3	30	30
Wed	weights	10	3	30	60
Fri	weights	10	3	30	90
				Total load	90

increasing in total load or tapering, whichever is appropriate, and to flag up any sudden increases or drops so that they can be examined for validity before you embark upon the training.

Table 15.7 Weight training load calculated by repetitions and resistance

Day	Lift	Reps	Sets	Total Reps	Resistance	Load	Load, running total
Mon	deadlift	10	3	30	70 kg	2100	2100
Wed	deadlift	10	3	30	70 kg	2100	4200
Fri	deadlift	10	3	30	75 kg	2250	6450
Mon	bench press	10	3	30	50 kg	1500	7950
Wed	bench press	10	3	30	55 kg	1650	9600
Fri	bench press	10	3	30	55 kg	1650	11,250
						Total load	11,250

In Figure 15.9 the hypothetical training year culminates in a competitive time in August when the intensity of training is at its peak and the volume of training is low. Immediately after the competition mesocycle the intensity of training drops, however volume is also relatively low at this point as active recovery takes place. The increase in volume then is shadowed by increases in intensity until volume drops to allow for high intensity training.

In this example load gradually increases and then drops in July and August during competition. September brings a recovery phase and then the load starts to rise again.

Date	Type of Exercise	Intensity	Time/Dur	Notes
07-Mar Fri	rest day			
08-Mar Sat	run	1–2	15 miles	easy
09-Mar Sun	bike	2	20 miles	steady
10-Mar Mon	run	2–2	12 miles	steady – somewhat hard
11-Mar Tue	run	3	6 reps	intervals
12-Mar Wed	run	2	14 miles	steady
13-Mar Thu	swim		30 mins	
14-Mar Fri	rest day	1		
15-Mar Sat	run	2	17 miles	easy
16-Mar Sun	bike	2	20 miles	steady
17-Mar Mon	run	2–3	6 miles	steady – somewhat hard
18–Mar Tue	run	3	8 reps	intervals
19–Mar Wed	run	1–2	17 miles	steady
21–Mar Fri	swim		30 mins	
22-Mar Sat	rest day			
23-Mar Sun	run	2–3	13 miles	half marathon RACE Fleet
24-Mar Mon	swim		30 mins	

Figure 15.8 Record of weekly total load

Many people believe that to lose body fat you must work aerobically and at low intensities. In fact losing body fat is a matter of creating a calorie deficit. It is a case of calories in versus calories out. To lose body fat you must expend more calories than you eat. How you do that is largely irrelevant. Thus you can work at high intensity for half an hour or at low intensity for one and a half hours; as long as the calorific requirement is the same the choice is yours. You can choose to mix weight training with cardiovascular training or you can choose to add in high intensity aerobic work or even plyometrics or sprinting, whatever you prefer.

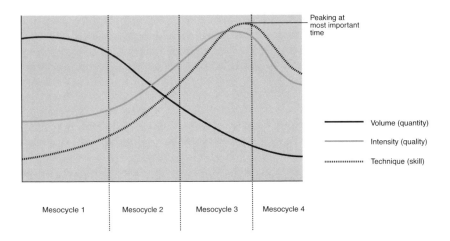

Fig 15.9 Changes in volume and intensity of training at different times of year (hypothetical)

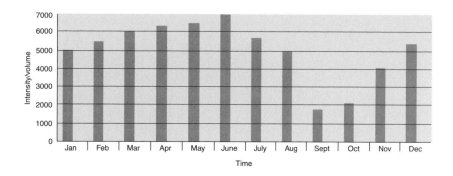

Figure 15.11 Example of annual training load

More than one way to skin a cat

It is possible to elicit the same physiological response by more than one method of training. For instance, training to raise anaerobic threshold can involve one continuous training session or interval training.

Similarly, in bodybuilding circles many people advocate a preferred method of training in order to gain maximum size or increased definition. Each proponent of each method can quote many examples of success as evidence that their favourite method works best.

Seeing the imbalance of musculature between the dominant and non-dominant arm in a tennis player or the dominant and non-dominant leg in a squash player; or seeing the muscular back of a rower, or the legs of a speed skater will provide evidence that heavy resistance training is not the only way to increase muscle bulk.

In summary, each individual is different and the training methods chosen rely on variations of FITT and are dependent on the physiological response, determined by assessing the limiting factor of performance and that person's individual response to training.

Progressive overload

Rest is an integral part of training. Many people forget that the harder you train, relatively speaking, the more you must rest to recover, relatively speaking. Exactly how much rest you need will partly depend on your training status and partly on your individual response to training. However, training too much in terms of volume, frequency or intensity leads to poor performance and eventually to overtraining syndrome and illness or injury.

> More training does not always mean better performance.

To avoid overtraining the principles of progressive overload should be followed. Increasing the volume or intensity of training too much will be detrimental to performance and might eventually lead to a chronic state of fatigue and to ill health. To ensure that this does not happen many individuals train by alternating one week hard, one week easy. Others work on two-week cycles. Some progressively overload for four or five weeks and then have an easy week.

> **Rule of thumb**
> Don't increase training by more than 10% per week.

Remember, overload can occur by increasing volume or intensity or both. The general stresses of daily life add to the stress of training and may increase the risk of overtraining. If you are working hard at a stressful job, suffering from lack of sleep

Microcycles				
22-Jul (7 weeks)	**skill**			
skill aerobic base/anaerobic recovery strength	skill training x 3 per week aerobic base - run/swim interval/fartlek runs weights			
29-Jul	**05-Aug**	**12-Aug**	**19-Aug**	**26 Aug**
swimming easy x 1 run x 1 steady state run x 1 anaerobic intervals weights x 2 skate training x 2	swimming easy x 1 run x 1 steady state run x 1 anaerobic intervals weights x 2 skate training x 2 swim tri	swimming easy x 1 run x 1 steady state run x 1 anaerobic intervals weights x 2 skate training x 2	easy week ultra fit rowing competition	swimming easy x 1 run x 1 steady state run x 1 anaerobic intervals weights x 2 skate training x 2

Figure 16.1 By planning mesocycles and microcycles it is simple to ensure that an easy week is regularly built into a programme

or lack of time to prepare food then you run a higher risk of becoming injured or overtrained.

An individual who is simply tired will, however, recover very quickly with a few days' rest, whereas overtraining syndrome is characterised by a sudden decline in performance that takes some time to remedy.

Tapering

Coming up to an event you need to reduce training levels, that is, you need taper. How long the taper is will depend on how long the event is. A long event will need a long taper. Some authors suggest as long as four weeks' taper for a marathon. It is best to taper the volume of training rather than the intensity.

06-Jan						Macrocycle							28-Apr		
January				February				March					April		
6	13	20	27	3	10	17	24	3	10	17	24	31	7	14	21	28

		Mesocycles		
06-Jan		03-Feb	03-Mar	07-Apr
				recovery

Microcycles				
03-Mar (5 weeks)				
03-Mar	10-Mar	17-Mar	24-Mar	31-Mar
7 days	7 days	7 days	7 days	7 days
steady run x 3	steady run x 3	steady run x 3	steady run x 3	taper week
interval run	interval run	interval run	interval run	
LSD x 1	LSD x 1	LSD x 1	LSD x 1	
bike 20 miles	bike 20 miles	bike 20 miles	bike 20 miles	
swim 30 mins	swim 30 mins	swim 30 mins	swim 30 mins	

Figure 16.2 Tapering before a race allows for full recovery from training sessions and replenishment of glycogen stores in preparation for the race

Overtraining syndrome

If overtraining continues it may progress to chronic stage. The signs of overtraining syndrome are:

• decline in performance;

• loss of muscle strength;

• loss of co-ordination;

• decline in maximal work capacity;

- decreased appetite;

- loss of weight;

- occasional nausea;

- muscle tenderness;

- minor infections;

- allergies;

- elevated resting heart rate;

- elevated blood pressure.

As you will see, many of these signs occur for other reasons. To complicate matters further, different individuals will respond differently to overtraining, not all will exhibit the same combination of symptoms nor in the same order of appearance.

Rule of thumb
The first sign of overtraining is usually decreased performance.

Other reliable indicators are heart rate and blood lactate responses to a standardised bout of training.

For instance, if a particular cycle ride normally takes you 30 minutes to complete with a heart rate of around 170 but starts taking 32 minutes with a heart rate of 175–180 this should alert you to look at your training and see if you are building in enough rest or if you are overloading too much. The same applies if your rate of perceived exertion goes up for a standardised training session.

Injury
Increasing the level of training too much also increases the risk of injury.

Injuries may be due to trauma, such as a fall or collision, or overuse.

Overuse injuries often occur when there is a sudden change within the training,

Rule of thumb
Change only one part of the training at a time.

such as a rapid increase in volume or intensity or when the training terrain is changed suddenly. Often injuries occur if too much of the training is changed at once, for instance adding in hill training, or weight training, or increasing the volume of training altogether.

R.I.C.E.
Treatment of injury is always RICE:

Rest the injured area
Ice or cool the injured area
Compression using a bandage or tubigrip
Elevation by raising the injured area up if possible to heart level.

If this first aid treatment is promptly applied and the help of a medical professional is promptly sought, most soft tissue injuries can be healed relatively quickly.

Problems usually occur when the athlete tries to work through the injury or pain.

Multi-sport training and injury

When injury occurs multi-sport training allows the athlete to continue training by working around the injury.

One client, a runner who sustained a stress fracture in the foot, continued training by cycling and swimming and found that he enjoyed it so much that he branched out into triathlon.

By using multi-sport training modes it is possible to maintain fitness whilst recovering from injury and also to use multi-sport training itself to aid with strengthening and flexibility work in order to rehabilitate fully. Even when using multi-sport training, however, progression to full training after injury should be gradual if injury is not to become recurrent.

17 The principles of training

Limiting factors to performance

In physiological terms there can only ever be one limiting factor to performance.

For instance, in the case of endurance sports, depending on the individual's training status, a different physiological adaptation is needed in order to improve performance. A beginner will make huge improvements by increasing cardiac output and thus MVO_2; however, an athlete who is training regularly may be limited by cellular adaptations and may make further improvements by improving the number and size of the capillaries supplying the working muscle and the number and size of the mitochondria in the muscle fibres. Therefore, whereas the beginner may well gain much from doing most training at 60–75 per cent of maximum heart rate, a more advanced performer will benefit from increasing the variety of the training intensities.

Physiological adaptations run along a continuum from low-intensity to high-intensity training. Whereabouts on the training continuum the physiological changes take place is partly dependent on the genetic inheritance and partly on the training status of the athlete. For instance, training at a heart rate equal to 85 per cent of MVO_2 will for one athlete be right on the limit of the anaerobic threshold and for another be below anaerobic threshold. For deconditioned individuals training at 60 per cent MVO_2 could be crossing the anaerobic threshold. To reach their potential most athletes will have to do some training at all levels. How much training is spent at different intensities depends on the demands of the sport and the limiting factor in the athlete's performance.

> For deconditioned individuals training at 60% MVO_2 could be crossing the anaerobic threshold.

The combination of intensity and duration of the stimulus placed upon skeletal muscle fibre changes the metabolic adaptations within them. For instance, sprinting relies on fast twitch fibres and on the anaerobic energy systems. Short sprint bursts, lasting less than 10 seconds but at maximal power rely heavily on the creatine phosphate system and on the high velocity of contraction of type IIb fibres. Lactic acid build-up interferes with the creatine phosphate system, and during training for sprint events the athletes aim to produce maximal power without building up lactic acid. They produce repeats of maximum effort for very short duration. This training may involve work intervals of maximum effort for 5–15 seconds followed by a long recovery period of 1–2 minutes such that the creatine phosphate is fully replenished and maximum effort can be repeated. This type of training produces optimum

Table 17.1 Adaptations that take place during training

	%MVO₂	%MHR	Adaptations	Energy systems	Fibre type recruitment
low intensity	55–65%	60–70%	Cardiovascular function Fluid balance Substrate availability	aerobic	slow twitch
	65–85%	70–90%	Cardiovascular function Mitochondrial density Capillary density	aerobic	type IIA
	85–100%	90–100%	Mitochondrial density Capillary density Lactate tolerance	anaerobic glycolysis	
	>100%	N/A	Maximum force generation Lactate tolerance	anaerobic glycolysis PCr	
high intensity					fast twitch

Note: the adaptations taking place during training are complex and multifaceted. This table suggests only towards which end of the continuum between low intensity and high intensity different energy systems predominate, fibre type recruitment takes place and adaptations may be assumed to occur.

recruitment of fibres for maximum force generation.

Middle distance events rely on fast twitch fibres and on anaerobic glycolysis to sustain a high power output for 2–3 minutes. Training the muscle to use glycogen in anaerobic pathways and to clear the lactate from the muscle more quickly is important. Thus these individuals may include high intensity intervals of 1–3 minutes alternated with recovery periods of 1–2 minutes such that lactate builds up in the muscle but a consistently high intensity is maintained throughout the training session.

Naturally, how much time you have available is of great importance. A common mistake when people start a new training programme is that in a burst of enthusiasm they plan to train more often than they can actually fit into their lifestyle. Failing to stick to the training programme can be very demotivating. I know of many people who have given up because they were unable to stick to the rigorous programme that they had set themselves and instead of simply downsizing the programme and their goals they stopped training all together.

Frequency refers to how often you train overall and also to how often at each intensity of exercise, so in a running programme, for instance, frequency refers to how often you run, how often you run on-road or off-road and how often you run at different intensities. If you multi-sport train by cycling, paddling, swimming, strength-training etc. as well, all these are added in as variables of frequency.

The frequency with which you train not only affects your adaptation to training but also your recovery from training sessions and your risk of injury or illness. The body adapts to unaccustomed stress, so you have to make it work harder and more often in order to adapt to that regime. Although there are benefits to even a single bout of exercise, many of the training adaptations take weeks of consistent training before they appear. Training too infrequently allows for retrogression to occur before the next training stimulus is applied and so no progress is made. To improve aerobic fitness you need to train at least three times per week. Training fewer times than this allows for retrogression to occur, offsetting the hard-earned improvements made to your physiology.

Similarly, if you train too often your body will not have enough time to adapt to the stresses that you place upon it. As well as training, the body needs rest in order to recuperate and to adapt.

Health guidelines suggest that we should do 30–60 minutes of moderate-intensity activity most days of the week in order to maintain or improve our health. Fitness guidelines suggest that we should do 20–30 minutes of vigorous aerobic activity three times a week plus two sessions of resistance-type training in order to maintain or improve fitness.

If your goals are performance-related these guidelines may not apply.

When training for a specific event it pays to remember the SAID principle (see box).

For instance, training to run or cycle distance must involve running or cycling distance; training to run or cycle fast must involve running or cycling fast. Training to run hills must involve running hills. Downhill running employs slightly different muscle fibres and in a different type of contraction to uphill running. Downhill running on a smooth surface is different from boulder-hopping down tracks on the fells. Off-road cycling involves different muscle activity from road cycling. Each of these employs and adapts the muscle fibres in slightly different physiological aspects.

SAID

SPECIFIC
ADAPTATION to
IMPOSED
DEMAND

In order, therefore, to train for a specific event the first principle is to look at the demands of that event and then start to simulate them.

Running a mountain marathon, for instance, involves two long days out on the fells carrying a pack. The terrain is rough and the weather often rougher, so training should involve as much fell running as possible and should involve at least one long steady run per week. Long, steady training for this event entails 3–4 hour training runs whereas training for a half marathon would involve 1–2 hour training runs.

When putting the programme together you should take into account the state of your fitness levels now and the time you have before your goal(s). Writing a training programme is a bit like fitting a jigsaw together.

More than one way to train

Every chain that breaks gives way at the point of its weakest link. If you strengthen or replace that weak link the chain will be stronger, but somewhere there will still be a weakest link. Keep adding stress and that new weakest link will eventually break.

It would seem that the key to improving performance lies in identifying the weakest link, creating physiological stresses that cause adaptation in that link and then maintaining that adaptation while working on the next weak link.

Each athlete, whether recreational or professional, has only one weakest link. Whether it be strength, cardiac output, ability to tolerate high levels of lactate, ability to work close to threshold for extended periods of time, flexibility, or whatever, there is always one aspect of physiology or biomechanics that limits performance. That weak link is individual to the athlete.

High versus low intensity?

Inevitably, to stress all aspects of physiology, at some time during training an athlete will work at high intensity and at some time will work at low intensity. High intensity work may be one continuous effort or may be as work–rest intervals.

Interval training – how it helps

If we increase all elements of training at once, that is frequency, intensity, and time or duration, we are likely to overtrain, thus it is beneficial to juggle these changes. An increase in intensity is normally accompanied by a decrease in total training volume so that the athlete does not become too fatigued.

As well as decreasing total training volume to facilitate the increase in intensity it is often necessary to reduce the time spent at that intensity. High-intensity exercise causes acute fatigue, often due to a depletion of the adenosine tri-phosphate (ATP) or creatine phosphate in the muscle, following a build-up of lactic acid. However, if the energy system that is taxed is allowed to recover the athlete may be able to repeat the effort at that same intensity, thus increasing the total volume of training time at the given high intensity.

Long-duration, **low-intensity** continuous exercise has been shown to improve performance in highly trained individuals; thus elite XC skiers in Norway train at around 60% of their VO_2max for about 80% of their training time. Huge improvements in performance times are widely documented for other elite endurance athletes, such as in running and cycling, after **high-intensity** training.

How is it possible to work hard for longer with intervals?

High-intensity work relies more on anaerobic energy systems and thus accumulates more lactic acid.

Let us suppose that John can cycle at 15 mph for a couple of hours, but at 20 mph can only manage ten minutes before he has to slow down. This is because at 20 mph John starts to rely more heavily on his anaerobic metabolism and gradually accumulates lactic acid. The lactic acid blocks muscle contraction and prevents him from maintaining his pace. He feels heavy-legged, and although he is trying even harder he cannot maintain 20 mph.

Now if John can easily cycle at 20 mph for just three minutes, he might feel fine and that he could continue, but in reality his muscles are already beginning to accumulate lactic acid. If, however, he drops his speed to 14–15 mph for the next three minutes, his body will clear the lactic acid from his muscles. He will now be able to cycle at 20 mph again for another three minutes. Working this way he might be able to achieve six to eight work intervals of three minutes at 20 mph, a total of 18–24 minutes at 20 mph as opposed to ten minutes at this higher intensity. Thus he has achieved a greater volume of training at a high intensity than if he tried to maintain 20 mph as steady state.

Can interval training help endurance athletes?

Altering the work–rest ratio and the intensity of both stresses different energy systems and recruits different fibre types. For instance, to increase aerobic capacity by affecting central circulation:

- you could train continuously for 20–40 minutes at around 70 per cent VO_2max,

- or you could train in 1.5-minute intervals with 1.5-minute rest at 85–90 per cent VO_2max.

The first method increases heart and ventilation rates and for the trained individual is unlikely to cause a build-up of lactic acid. The second method increases heart and ventilation rates, and if continued for a longer period of time would be limited by build-up of lactic acid, but in short bursts is enough to elicit the central response whilst allowing enough recovery time to clear the lactate. However, the second method, being of higher intensity will recruit more of the fast twitch fibres.

Which is best, interval training or continuous exercise?

As always, the answer is, 'That depends!' It depends on the aim of the training session. To get the best from our training we sometimes need to work at low and sometimes at high intensities. When working at high intensities it is often possible to increase the overall workload; that is, to work for longer at that intensity, by using interval training.

The science of interval training

A *Textbook of Work Physiology* by Per Olaf Astrand and Kaare Rodahl reports Dr Astrand's renowned study on the physiology of continuous exercise versus intermittent exercise or interval training.[1] Dr Astrand studied subjects who had to achieve a given amount of work in one hour. The work was carried out either by cycling continuously at a power output of 175 watts, or at intervals with a power output of 350 watts – that is, double the power output (see table 18.1). If the same

Table 18.1 Continuous versus interval training

At a workload of 175 watts,	At a workload of 350 watts
• The subject was able to cycle for one hour continuously	• The subject could only maintain one the exercise for 9 min
• Heart rate was 134bpm	• Heart rate reached 190bpm
• VO_2 was 55% of maximal	• VO_2 was at max
• Blood lactate remained near resting levels	• Blood lactate had risen to 16.5 **mM**

subject cycled at 350 watts for work intervals of between 30 seconds and 3 minutes with equal rest intervals, he could perform the desired workload within the hour.

Astrand's results clearly demonstrated that interval training allows a higher total volume of high intensity work to be performed than does continuous exercise. When working continuously the subject could achieve only 9 minutes at 350 watts while when working in intervals he could continue for 30 minutes.

mM = mMols, a measure of blood lactate measured in mMols per litre. Anaerobic threshold is normally said to be at 4.0 mM/l.

How long should the intervals be?

Interestingly, the physiological responses differ depending on the interval duration; when the work intervals are shortened, the physiological stress is reduced. In fact, even though the total work time and work intensity are kept the same when the intervals are reduced to less than 2 minutes, the physiological stress is much reduced as signified by the VO_2, the heart rate and accumulated blood lactate in table 18.2.

So, is this good?

The greater total volume of training at higher intensity puts a greater workload on the muscles, but the effect that it has on the heart and central circulation depends on the length of the work/rest intervals. It is thought that during very brief intervals the build-up of lactate is reduced because the muscles utilise the oxygen that is bound to the myoglobin in the muscle cells for aerobic energy production. The recovery phase allows for the myoglobin oxygen stores to be replenished, thus the demand made on the oxygen delivery system is not severe. However when the work interval is

Table 18.2 *Astrand's study of the effects of continuous and intermittent high-intensity exercise*

Power output	Exercise condition	VO_2 l/min	Heart rate acid mM	Blood lactic
175 watts	Continuous	2.44	134	1.3
350 watts	Continuous	4.6	190	16.5
350 watts	Intermittent 30 sec	2.90	150	2.2
350 watts	Intermittent 1 min	2.93	167	5.0
350 watts	Intermittent 2 min	4.4	178	10.5
350 watts	Intermittent 3 min	4.6	188	13.2

* Rest duration equalled work duration in each condition.

increased in length the myoglobin oxygen stores are depleted without subsequent replenishment during recovery periods. This results in a greater demand being made on the cardiovascular system and greater build-up of lactic acid.

By greatly shortening the work and rest periods, even as far as to 15 seconds of work and 15 seconds of rest, it is possible to perform at very high power outputs without accumulating lactic acid or severely stressing the cardiovascular system.[2] Thus it is possible, by using interval training with short intervals, less than say two minutes in length, to put an increased workload on the muscle fibres. If recruitment of fibres and demand on aerobic metabolism in the muscle cells is the aim of the session this would appear to work.

Interval training for improved central circulation

By increasing the length of the intervals to a point where the demand on the oxygen delivery system is greater, it is possible to elevate the heart rate and overload the capacity of the heart to pump blood around the body. The body's response to this is to adapt such that it increases cardiac output and stroke volume and thus pumps out more blood with each beat. Of course, continuous training at high intensity will also have this effect; however, with continuous high-intensity training a build-up of lactate causes local muscle fatigue and limits the time spent at the increased cardiac output. Interval training allows the lactate to disperse and so increases the total time spent at the increased cardiac output.

Should deconditioned individuals do interval training?

As you can see, by playing with work–rest intervals and intensity of effort the physiological stress can be reduced. Beginners to exercise can in this way obtain health benefits from training their heart and circulation by working intervals. The

Intervals can be of any intensity. The work rest period can be:

work
low intensity

rest
lower intensity

rather than:

work
high intensity

rest
low intensity

stress experienced is less and so the total workload is greater if they slow down or stop before becoming too uncomfortable, and then start again.

How do I split up the intervals?

How you split the intervals depends on what you want to achieve and can tolerate. Often enthusiastic sports participants try to follow the training programme of a top-level athlete who is both genetically gifted and able to dedicate large portions of her or his life to training and resting. How much training a person can tolerate, the dosage in which they can tolerate it and their response to it are influenced by genetic coding, lifestyle, training history and age.

For instance, working at level 4 for 3-minute intervals with a 3-minute rest may give one athlete just enough recovery time to be able to repeat the work interval at the same intensity for ten repetitions. Another athlete may need to achieve five of the intervals, have a longer rest period, say six minutes, and then repeat the set. Each athlete achieves 10 x 3-minute intervals; however, one athlete achieves this in one set of ten and the other athlete in two sets of five.

Writing a training programme is an art directed but not ruled by science. Each athlete must be treated as an individual: what works for one person may not work for the next. The splitting of intervals is therefore a matter of looking at the physiological changes that you want to affect by the training, the intensity at which those intervals will be attempted and the athlete's present capabilities.

The fibre type you wish to recruit and the energy system you wish to tax will determine the work–rest periods.

Table 18.3 Guidelines for interval times for training different energy systems

	Type	Work time	Rest time
Steady state	continuous	30–60 min	
Anaerobic threshold	continuous	15–25 min	
Anaerobic threshold	intervals	60–90 sec	10–15 sec
Lactate tolerance	intervals	60–180 sec	60–120 sec
Anaerobic alactic	intervals	5–15 sec	60–120 sec

Sprint training

Short bursts of power as in sprinting and weightlifting rely on the fast twitch fibres and the ATP supplies and creatine phosphate systems. As lactic acid interferes with the creatine phosphate system the work intervals for this type of training should be short and the rest intervals long; work intervals of 5–15 seconds are alternated with rest intervals of 1–2 minutes, so that the work time is not long enough to build up lactic acid and a full recovery of the creatine phosphate system is facilitated.

The energy supply used in this type of interval work is sometimes termed 'anaerobic alactic' as it is anaerobic but does not involve build up of lactic acid.

Lactate tolerance

Work intervals of 1–3 minutes alternated with 1–2 minutes' rest also stress the anaerobic energy systems. The work interval is long enough to build up lactic acid and this type of training is often called 'lactate tolerance'. In reality, rather than training the muscles to tolerate high levels of lactate the muscles become efficient at flushing the lactate into the bloodstream, which enables them to keep working at high intensities.

Anaerobic threshold

Intervals of 1–1.5 minutes of work alternated with 10–15 seconds' rest raises the anaerobic threshold or point of onset of blood lactate accumulation (OBLA). Continuous training at an intensity that allows you to sustain one continuous effort of 15–25 minutes has the same effect. Raising the anaerobic threshold will allow you to sustain work at higher intensities using aerobic metabolism. In other words, the result of this training is that you perform faster for longer.

Steady state

Steady state training uses the aerobic system, and trains for improved VO_2max and utilisation of fats.

19 Fitting the jigsaw together

If you are multi-sport training just to add variety to your fitness programme, then structuring it very carefully is less important than if you multi-sport train within a goal-oriented programme, such as aiming to perform in a particular sporting event.

However, even if you are simply adding variety to your programme, adding structure may be useful to ensure that you do not get stuck in a rut.

Sporting events

Within sports distinct seasons can be identified and different types of training can be written into a programme that respects these seasons. To get the best out of the programme it needs structure. One way of structuring is to use a technique known as 'periodisation' (see also chapter 15). Periodisation is a programming technique developed in training for sports performance. However, it lends a sound framework to writing a training programme that can be used for any purpose, be it for a sports performer, or fitness enthusiast. It provides a way of ensuring that you gain maximum benefits for minimum risk and that you achieve whatever realistic goals you may have set.

05-Oct					Macrocycle						25-Oct	
Oct	Nov	Dec	Jan	Feb	Mar	Apr	May	Jun	Jul	Aug	Sep	Oct

5 12 19 26 2 9 16 23 30 7 14 21 28 4 11 18 25 1 8 15 22 29 1 8 15 22 29 5 12 19 26 3 10 17 24 31 7 14 21 28 5 12 19 26 2 9 16 23 30 6 13 20 27 4 11 18 25

Figure 19.1 The macrocycle

First you identify a main period of time culminating in a major goal or sporting event. This period of time is called a 'macrocycle' (figure 19.1). It may be a complete year or may be more than or less than a year in time. You then divide the macrocycle up into shorter time phases, each having a purpose such as to build strength, increase skill or improve speed.

Within training for competitive sport there are four distinct and ordered phases of training called 'mesocycles'. They are conditioning, preparation, competition and recovery.

Dividing the macrocycle into mesocycles assists with the in-depth planning of the preparation and training needed to achieve (or be ready for) the goal.

Each mesocycle does not have to be the same length but clearly they must all add up to the length of the macrocycle.

Within sports performance each mesocycle is a distinct phase of training that

127

aims to achieve specific adaptations. Thus a competitive sprinter may spend his conditioning mesocycle building strength and power, and his preparation mesocycle adding speed, reaction time and the will to win. A marathon runner may spend his conditioning phase building endurance and his preparation time increasing his overall speed over long distances.

Aims for each mesocycle can then be added to the programme (figure 19.2).

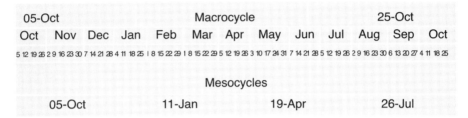

Figure 19.2 Added aims for each mesocycle

If you are training just for fun then each individual mesocycle may focus on a different main sport or a different set of sports. For instance in the summer your mesocycles may focus on cycling and climbing and in winter on swimming and weight training.

The mesocycles are further split into 'microcycles' (figure 19.3). Each microcycle consists of a number of days of training. Typically each microcycle covers a week, though it could be shorter or longer. Each is planned with a particular training adaptation in mind, and takes into account the workload of the previous and the following microcycles.

The whole programme then is planned and designed with a top-down approach. The details of the programme depend on:

• goals;

• present level of training and experience;

• time available for training;

• necessary training adaptations;

• ability to sustain a planned level of training.

Planning your programme

To plan your programme, therefore, you must:

1 Look at your long-term goals. Perhaps they are to run a half marathon, cycle in a ten-mile fun or 100-mile Audax ride, swim in a gala in the 400-metre freestyle, or compete in a triathlon; or they may be things such as losing or gaining weight, reducing your blood pressure, or being fit enough to enjoy your skiing holiday.

2 Identify the length of time in which you wish to achieve the goal. This is your macrocycle.

3 Identify subgoals. These may be things such as to compete in a shorter race than that chosen as your main goal, or to make improvements in time for a distance that

05-Oct						Macrocycle					25-Oct	
Oct	Nov	Dec	Jan	Feb	Mar	Apr	May	Jun	Jul	Aug	Sep	Oct

5 12 19 26 29 16 23 30 7 14 21 28 4 11 18 25 | 8 15 22 29 | 8 15 22 29 5 12 19 26 3 10 17 24 31 7 14 21 28 5 12 19 26 29 16 23 30 6 13 20 27 4 11 18 25

Mesocycles			
05-Oct	11-Jan	19-Apr	26-Jul
1	2	3	4

Microcycles	
11-Jan (4 weeks)	2

Conditioning	when elements such as strength and endurance are trained			
11-Jan	18-Jan	25-Jan	01-Feb	08-Feb
7 days	7 days	7 days	7 days	7 days

Figure 19.3 The microcycle

you already know that you can complete, or they might include improving your time around a training run, or running more often per week or increasing the weight you can lift for a particular set of repetitions.

4 Identify the training needs to achieve the main goals and subgoals. So, for instance, if you intend to cycle from John O'Groats to Lands End, the training need for a minigoal could be to be able to cycle for 100 miles in one day. If, however, the goal is to run a 5-kilometre race, the goal may be to be able to run 5 kilometres, or may be to put in speed sessions in order to be able to run it faster. Trying to improve all training needs at once is not necessarily the most effective way of achieving goals, so it helps to put the development of these in order of priority and of training principles. Thus if you want to run 5 kilometres faster than last year, but also to now run 10 kilometres, you may prioritise building up your distance to be able to run 10 K and then add in speed work to allow you to run 5 kilometres faster.

5 Split the macrocycle into mesocycles each devoted to the development of a training need. Document these phases so that each individual training need is worked on in turn, while maintaining that which has already been achieved. You will need to decide an appropriate timescale for each phase. Note that the phases can be of different lengths. The timescale for each phase will depend on:

• the sub-goals for that phase;

• the degree of physiological stress in that phase;

• your experience and fitness level;

• the time you have available to train on a weekly basis.

Having done all this you will need to make regular changes to the programme, accommodating:

- A recovery phase for the body by working on different aspects of fitness (this can be a phase where you train using a completely different sport);

- maintenance of interest in the programme (again, multi-sport training to add variety will help with this);

- continued adaptation by regularly changing the component of fitness being stressed.

6 Write the training instructions of each phase or mesocycle.
7 Take each phase or mesocycle and insert the microcycles (usually in weeks).
8 Write the individual workouts.

Having decided on the aim of each microcycle or week you can decide on the individual training sessions or workouts and write the details of those sessions. This allows you to plan precisely what you need to achieve in terms of intensity and volume.

Training volume

The body adapts only to unaccustomed stress. You should plan to increase the workload gradually in order to progress. Ideally you should plan to have an easy week every fourth or fifth week, so for three or four weeks the training level increases and then you have a recovery week. This allows your body to recoup and adapt from the previous increases in workload.

The workload or volume of training is a mixture of time and intensity. On days when you are training at high intensity the time should be reduced. On days when you are putting in a long session the intensity should be reduced. You can estimate a rough guide to training volume by:

- allocating a number to the intensity, either using a percentage effort or a perceived exertion scale or heart rate;

- allocating a number to the time using minutes;

- multiplying the intensity by the time to get an estimate of volume, (by doing this you can see whether volume is increasing or decreasing);

- adding together the volumes per day for a whole microcycle or week (you can then compare weeks to see if volume is increasing or decreasing as the programme progresses).

Session Plan

Date	Type of Exercise	Intensity	Time/Dur	Notes	Volume
01-Dec Mon	run	2	45 mins		
02-Dec Tue	run	4	8 mins	4 x 2 intervals	
03-Dec Wed	run	1–2	75 mins	long steady	
04-Dec Thu	rest day				
05-Dec Fri	run	2	45 mins		
06-Dec Sat	run	3	15 mins	thershold session	
07-Dec Sun	run	2	40 mins		412
08-Dec Mon	run	2	45 mins		
09-Dec Tue	run	4	10 mins	4 x 2 intervals	
10-Dec Wed	run	1–2	85 mins	long steady	
11-Dec Thu	rest day				
12-Dec Fri	run	2	50 mins		
13-Dec Sat	run	3	15 mins	thershold session	
14-Dec Sun	run	2	40 mins		440
15-Dec Mon	run	2	45 mins		
16-Dec Tue	run	4	10 mins	4 x 2 intervals	
17-Dec Wed	run	1–2	90 mins	long steady	
18-Dec Thu	rest day				
19-Dec Fri	run	2	60 mins		
20-Dec Sat	run	3	15 mins	thershold session	
21-Dec Sun	run	2	40 mins		465
22-Dec Mon	run	2	45 mins		
23-Dec Tue	run	4	8 mins	4 x 2 intervals	
24-Dec Wed	run	1–2	90 mins	long steady	
25-Dec Thu	rest day				

Figure 19.4 Calculating the training volume; the weekly training volume is calculated by multiplying intensity by time

Programmes for different types of athlete

Single sports

Single-sport athletes need to determine why they are multi-sport training, and then vary the training depending on which mesocycle they are in. For these athletes, multi-sport training may not be appropriate all the year round.

Research clearly shows that for single-sport athletes nearing their genetic ceiling for performance, multi-sport training is not the best way to find the tiny increments in performance that make the difference between winning or coming second. For sports performers multi-sport training programmes that are designed without regard for the primary sport may actually increase the incidence of injury.[1] Indeed, even in untrained individuals, the aerobic benefits from a single sport are the same as those from multi-sport training given similar volume and intensity of training.[2]

It may be that they multi-sport train during active rest, working the body while resting the mind. It may be that they multi-sport train only during the off-season, to build on baseline fitness parameters such as flexibility, aerobic power or strength, or

The National Collegiate Athletic Association (NCAA) has gathered statistics over a three-year period in the early 1990s showing that women suffered anterior cruciate ligament injuries more often than men, nearly four times as often in basketball, three times as often in gymnastics, and nearly two and a half times as often in soccer.

Many factors have been discussed as the source of women's tendency to tear their ACL more often. Some are based on anatomical realities such as a narrower femoral notch, increased Q angle, increased ligamentous laxity, inadequate strength, and impaired neuromuscular co-ordination.

Strength training for women is critical, with an emphasis on being in shape before they play their sport. Women tend to be generally more flexible than men, but a programme that consists of strengthening and stretching is essential for all athletes involved in sports. Non-competitive balance and agility training may enhance proprioceptive function and help to reduce the rate of injury as well.

NISMAT website Hot Topics Page on Knee Injuries and the Female Athlete
http://www.nismat.org/hot

to alter muscular imbalances that negatively affect technique in their sport; but then focus should switch to the individual sport as the competitive season gets closer. It may be that they multi-sport train when rehabilitating from injury in order to maintain high levels of fitness without aggravating the injury. It may be that they multi-sport train throughout the season to correct or maintain muscular balance and avoid recurrence of injury.

Whatever the reason for multi-sport training, the single sport athlete must keep their primary goal in mind.

Case study

A client of mine who lived in London was a mountain marathoner. His sport was orienteering competitions run over two days somewhere in the mountains of the United Kingdom or Europe. He typically travelled 25 to 30 kilometres over rough hilly country with few if any footpaths on each day of competition. Often the weather was stormy and throughout the competition he carried provisions for the two days and for an overnight camp on the hills in bad weather.

As he lived in central London, sport-specific training, running on the hills with a pack, was only possible when he could get a couple of day-trips to the hills, so much of his training had to be a compromise. At one time he plodded the streets of London with a pack; however, he found that London streets were too busy to allow him to keep moving and the extra weight of his pack increased the impact on his joints which, when pavement plodding, predisposed him to knee injury. He tried running on a treadmill at an incline with his pack, which was an improvement, but he got very hot running indoors with a pack and also he found it slightly embarrassing to run with a pack on his back in a club.

> Note that downhill running works the eccentric contraction of the leg muscles especially the quadriceps (thighs), thus by strengthening this phase using the downward motion involved in squats and lunges eccentric strength is trained. This will benefit the athlete in stabilising the knee joint during downhill running. Free weights are better than fixed resistance in this instance as they also use other fixator muscles simulating fixation when running with a pack.

Finally, he decided to seek help. We structured his training programme to include weight training to build up upper body strength so that he suffered less upper body fatigue during the event. We also included lower body work with free weights (deadlift, squats and lunges) so that he had the strength to keep his joints in alignment during both uphill and downhill running over rough country. The weight training improved and maintained strength enough to allow him to reduce the amount of time he spent running with a pack, and in fact he no longer ran with a pack when running on pavements or on the treadmill. We added intervals and hill work on the treadmill and circuit training, which added agility and power work. This was to help with balance on the rough ground and ability to descend quickly, and he started to cycle to and from work for extra endurance training without extra impact on the joints. At weekends he travelled out of London into Epping Forest or onto the North Downs (about an hour's travel time each way) as often as possible and this provided some rougher country to train on. Nearer to the time of his events he increased his trips to the hills for specific training. On his weekend trips he ran with a pack.

He found that because he was adding in more variety of training he did not get stale, but trained more and harder. Not only did his performance in mountain marathon improve, but also, because of the variety and the improvement in his fitness levels, he found it easier to motivate himself to train.

05-Jan			Macrocycle			29-Jun
January	February		March	April	May	June
5 12 19 26	2 9 16 23		2 9 16 23 30	6 13 20 27	4 11 18 25	1 8 15 22 29

Mesocycles

05-Jan	16-Feb	06-Apr	25-May
base 1	base 2	build up	pre competition
endurance and strength	increase threshold and specific strength/endurance	power and endurance	specificity and taper for competition
add in weights. increase run distance gradually introduce and increase cycle to and from work	add hill running and intervals increase distance on some long runs, increase run training on rough country keep weights going add more free weights for lower body	add in circuits for agility and power keep weights going increase no of reps increase running intensity	more specific running with a pack over mountainous country. last two weeks taper for competition

Figure 20.1 Sample of multi-sport training programme for mountain marathon athlete

For the single-sport athlete multi-sport training activities aimed at the same physiological changes may improve performance, depending on the multi-sport training activity involved. For example, UK sports coach and sports physiologist Tony Lycholat noticed that runners who took up road cycling during rehabilitation from injury reported improvements in performance, but for runners who used a rowing ergometer during rehabilitation performance levels deteriorated. He surmised that the reason for this was that the speed of joint movement, utilisation of energy systems and velocity of contraction of fibres in spinning the pedals on a bike caused similar physiological stress to performance running, whereas the slow cadence of row training, normally less than 30 strokes per minute, placed different physiological stress on the body and therefore elicited a different adaptive response.

It would seem sensible then that a single-sport athlete using cross training as part of a training programme should choose disciplines that closely mimic fibre type recruitment, energy system utilisation and speed of movement of the primary sport.

Nevertheless, this many single-sport athletes may have other, perfectly sound reasons for cross training using non-compatible disciplines. If athlete's strength is the weak link in performance then he or she might well choose weight training. If

04-Sep	Macrocycle		26-Aug

Sep	Oct	Nov	Dec	Jan	Feb	Mar	Apr	May	Jun	Jul	Aug
4 11 18 25	2 9 16 23 30	6 13 20 27	4 11 18 25	1 8 15 22 29	5 12 19 26	4 11 18 25	1 8 15 22 29	6 13 20 27	3 10 17 24	1 8 15 22 29	5 12 19 26

Mesocycles		
04-Sep	15-Jan	06-May
conditioning	preparation	competition
strength specific to hills	anaerobic endurance	peak towards the main goal
increased threshold level	speed and power	sprint off the line
strength work 3 times per week	sprint work (intervals)	using competition as high
interval and threshold training	hill reps	intensity training
circuit X 2 per week – inclusive	weights once per week	Reaction training, sprint off
of rowing work.	plyometrics	the line.
plyometric towards end of		Ladies tolerance training
microcycle		

Figure 20.2 The mountain biker whose programme this is multi-sport trains with circuit and weight training and indoor rowing in his condition mesocycle; he drops the rowing in his preparation cycle and has a long competitive mesocycle in which he only cycles. In this phase he does low- and moderate-intensity cycling during training sessions and uses races as high-intensity training sessions. He will, however, taper for the National Championships in August and following them have a recovery phase

reaction time is the weak link, the athlete might play table tennis.

The recreational athlete

For recreational athletes the same applies, they may multi-sport train to alter muscle imbalances, to recover from injury or simply as a change from single-sport activity.

If they multi-sport train they approach it with more enthusiasm because of the variety, so training increases and they improve in their sport simply because the volume of training is higher.

Rule of thumb
Training should proceed according to the needs of the individual athlete. Each individual has one weak link. That weak link prevents them from improving. Train to strengthen the weak link and then look for the next weak link.

The fitness athlete

With the widespread popularity of health clubs and gyms containing a mix of cardiovascular and weights equipment, a new breed of sportsperson has emerged. Such a person often presents the trainer with a significant challenge in that he or she wants to achieve apparently totally incompatible goals, for instance: 'I want to build muscle and run a marathon'.

This fitness athlete whose goals these were wanted to build muscle, however he

Table 20.1 Multi-sport training plan for recreational marathon runner

Week	Mon	Tue	Wed	Thur	Fri	Sat	Sun	Total run
1	X20	5S	X20	6S	R	8S	11S	30
2	3F	4S	X25	8S	5F	R	13S	33
3	X25	3F	X30	6F	6F	R	15S	30
4	X35	6S	X40	8S	6F	R	15S	35
5	X40	5S	X45	3F	5F	R	17S	30
6	X50	8S	X55	5F	X55	R	20S	33
7	X60	3F	4F	10S	X60	R	18S	35
8	3F	3S	R	3F	R	R	**MARATHON**	35

R = Rest day, with stretching exercises
X = Cross train, e.g. swim or cycle; number denotes time in minutes
F = fast run; number denotes mileage
S = Slow run. Number denotes mileage

also wanted to compete in a triathlon and a 10-kilometre run. Thus rather than following the traditional mesocycle phasing his programme is aimed at building bulk with phases of increased endurance training designed to complete his endurance goals without losing too much of his hard-earned muscle (see figures

Date	Type of Exercise	Intensity	Time/Dur	Notes	
03-Feb Mon	run	2	3 miles	steady	
04-Feb Tue	run	3	3 reps	intervals	
05-Feb Wed	run	2	5 miles	steady	
06-Feb Thu	swim		30 mins		
07-Feb Fri	rest day				
08-Feb Sat	run	1–2	12 miles	easy pace	
09-Feb Sun	bike	1–2	20 miles	steady	57
10-Feb Mon	run	2	6 miles	intervals	
11-Feb Tue	run	3	4 reps	steady	
12-Feb Wed	bike	2	20 miles		
13-Feb Thu	run	1–2	12 miles		
14-Feb Fri	swim		30 mins		
16-Feb Sun	run	3	6 miles	10k RACE	
17-Feb Mon	run	2	4 miles	easy	94
18-Feb Tue	run	3	5 reps	intervals	
19-Feb Wed	bike		15 miles		
20-Feb Thu	run	2	8 miles	steady	

Figure 20.3 Section of multi-sport training plan for recreational runner using cycling and swimming

20.4 and 20.5).

To accommodate the competitive nature of this new breed of sportsperson gym-based multi-sport training challenges such as the Ultrafit challenge and TV Gladiators have grown up. Such challenges are generally a mixture of strength and

Macrocycle																			
August				September				October					November				December		
7	14	21	28	4	11	18	25	2	9	16	23	30	6	13	20	27	4	11	18	25

Mesocycles				
07-Aug	21-Aug	11-Sep	02-Oct	20-Nov
hypertrophy	hypertrophy	strength & run	run	hypertrophy
increase	increase muscle bulk	build on absolute strength	specific for ten k run endurance speed	increase muscle bulk
build up volume and intensity intensity of weights	build up volume and intensity of weights	increase intensity and decrease volume of weights. keep endurance steady	reduce weights to minimum, work on speed	increase volume of weights whilst maintaining high
endurance	endurance work moderate volume		last week active rest	endurance work, low volume, low intensity

Figure 20.4

Macrocycle																			
August				September				October					November				December		
7	14	21	28	4	11	18	25	2	9	16	23	30	6	13	20	27	4	11	18	25

Mesocycles				
07-Aug	21-Aug	11-Sep	02-Oct	20-Nov
hypertrophy	hypertrophy	strength & run	run	hypertrophy

Microcycles	
02-Oct (7 weeks)	run
specific for ten k run endurance speed	reduce weight to minimum, work on speed last week active rest

02-Oct	09-Oct	16-Oct	23-Oct	30-Oct
7 days	7 days	7 days	7 days	7 days
3 weight sessions, 2 day split. legs and arms, back and chest.	4 run sesions two steady one interval one threshold	4 run sessions 2 steady one interval one threshold	3 run sessions tapering distance maintaining speed one race	easy week 2 easy runs
3 runs, increase length. add one threshold	weights x 2 working on strength maintainance 2 day split	weights x 2 working on strength maintainance 2 day split	weights x 1 working on strength maintainance full body	weights x 2 working on strength 2 day split

Figure 20.5

endurance, speed and agility. Best results will be obtained when training is imaginative and is linked with a sound understanding of physiology so that the training programme will assist the fitness athlete in achieving the desired results. If

<table>
<tr><td colspan="9" align="center">Macrocycle</td></tr>
<tr><td>April</td><td>May</td><td>Jun</td><td>Jul</td><td>Aug</td><td>Sep</td><td>Oct</td><td>Nov</td><td></td></tr>
<tr><td colspan="9">7 14 21 28 5 12 19 26 2 9 16 23 30 7 14 21 28 4 11 18 25 1 8 15 22 29 6 13 20 27 3 10 17 24</td></tr>
</table>

Mesocycles				
07-Apr	23-Jun	04-Aug	01-Sep	06-Oct
phase 1	phase 2	australia	sport specific	competitive
strength and endurance	raised threshold increased power		sport specific	sport specific
increase strength and endurance on bike/row and run. VO2 max training and LSD short intervals	long intervals and threshold training. LSD up vertical power circuits		row long intervals long sprints	row power overspeed taper

Figure 20.6 In the macrocycle illustrated here the athlete has two mountain bike challenges, a mountain marathon and an indoor rowing championship. In the middle of the macrocycle he has planned a month's trip to Australia, for scuba diving

<table>
<tr><td colspan="9" align="center">Macrocycle</td></tr>
<tr><td>April</td><td>May</td><td>Jun</td><td>Jul</td><td>Aug</td><td>Sep</td><td>Oct</td><td>Nov</td><td></td></tr>
<tr><td colspan="9">7 14 21 28 5 12 19 26 2 9 16 23 30 7 14 21 28 4 11 18 25 1 8 15 22 29 6 13 20 27 3 10 17 24</td></tr>
</table>

Mesocycles				
07-Apr	23-Jun	04-Aug	01-Sep	06-Oct
phase 1	phase 2	australia	sport specific	competitive

Microcycles

07-Apr (11 weeks) — phase 1
strength and endurance — increase strength and endurance on bike/row and run. VO2 max training and LSD short intervals

07-Apr	14-Apr	21-Apr	28-Apr	05-May
7 days	7 days	7 days	7 days	7 days
	BIKE x 1 LSD, 1 short ints, 2 easy, 1 hard.: RUN x 1 steady, 1 short ints.: WEIGHTS x 1 strength ROW x 1 CIRCUITS x 2	BIKE x 1 LSD, 1 short ints, 2 easy, 1 hard.: RUN x 1 steady, 1 short ints.: WEIGHTS x 1 strength ROW x 1 CIRCUITS x 2	BIKE x 1 LSD, 1 short ints, 2 easy, 1 hard.: RUN x 1 steady, 1 short ints.: WEIGHTS x 1 strength ROW x 1 CIRCUITS x 2	BIKE x 1 LSD, 1 short ints, 2 easy, 1 hard.: RUN x 1 steady, 1 short ints.: WEIGHTS x 1 strength ROW x 1 CIRCUITS x 2

Figure 20.7 The athlete has five mescocycles, the first concentrating on strength and endurance. Towards the end of this mesocycle is his first major challenge, a two-day mountain bike competition

Macrocycle

April	May	Jun	Jul	Aug	Sep	Oct	Nov
7 14 21 28	5 12 19 26	2 9 16 23 30	7 14 21 28	4 11 18 25	1 8 15 22 29	6 13 20 27	3 10 17 24

Mesocycles

07-Apr	23-Jun	04-Aug	01-Sep	06-Oct
phase 1	phase 2	australia	sport specific	competitive

Microcycles

23-Jun (6 weeks)	phase 2
raised threshold and increased power	long intervals and threshold training. LSD Up vertical power circuits

23-Jun	30-Jun	07-Jul	14-Jul	21-Jul
7 days	7 days	7 days	7 days	7 days
BIKE x 1 LSD	BIKE x 1 LSD.	BIKE x 1 LSD.	BIKE x 1 LSD.	BIKE x 1 LSD.
1 threshold.	1 threshold	1 threshold	1 threshold	1 threshold
1 hills, others steady:	1 hills, others steady	1 hills, others steady	1 hills, others steady	1 hills, others steady
RUN x 1 LSD,	RUN x 1 LSD,	RUN x 1 LSD,	RUN x 1 LSD,	RUN x 1 LSD,
1 steady, 1 hills.:	1 steady, 1 hills.:	1 steady, 1 hills.:	1 steady, 1 hills.:	1 steady, 1 hills.:
WEIGHTS x 2 power	WEIGHTS x 2 power	WEIGHTS x 2 power	WEIGHTS x 2 power	WEIGHTS x 2 power
ROW x 1 steady,	ROW x 1 steady,	ROW x 1 steady,	ROW x 1 steady,	ROW x 1 steady,
1 intervals.:	1 intervals.:	1 intervals.:	1 intervals.:	1 intervals.:
CIRCUITS x 2	CIRCUITS x 2	CIRCUITS x 2	CIRCUITS x 2	CIRCUITS x 2

Figure 20.8 In the second mesocycle the athlete concentrates on increasing power and anaerobic threshold. During his trip to Australia he will attempt to keep up enough short-duration, high-intensity training to maintain these adaptions

you are one of these sportspeople, a good personal trainer should be able to help you.

Sometimes such multi-sports individuals simply have a number of different sports that they are keen to compete in. The competitions may be in different disciplines but each is a separate event. The athlete whose programme appears at figures 20.6 to 20.9 at various times competes in 10-kilometre and half-marathon road races, mountain marathons, indoor rowing competitions, mountain biking and gym-based challenges, as well as completing non-competitive, ultra-distance outdoor challenges.

Multi-sports

Multi-sports are, by definition, competitive multi-sport training events. However, as for single-sport events the athlete must focus on the needs of the sport. Often multidiscipline events such as pentathlon, heptathlon, or decathlon require considerable skill in a number of the disciplines, such as javelin throwing, jumping events and hurdling in the heptathlon and decathlon. As well as the technique training involved there is the combination of different types of fitness for different events, and the mental toughness to train for all of them – the athlete is often required to spend the most training time on improving his or her least-favourite discipline. Multi-sport athletes who combine events in this way are remarkable and dedicated people.

Macrocycle

April	May	Jun	Jul	Aug	Sep	Oct	Nov
7 14 21 28	5 12 19 26	2 9 16 23 30	7 14 21 28	4 11 18 25	1 8 15 22 29	6 13 20 27	3 10 17 24

Mesocycles

07-Apr		23-Jun	04-Aug	01-Sep	06-Oct
phase 1		phase 2	australia	sport specific	competitive

Microcycles

06-Oct (8 weeks)	competitive
sports specific	row power overspeed taper

27-Oct	03-Nov	10-Nov	17-Nov	24-Nov
7 days	7 days	7 days	7 days	7 days
BIKE x 1 hills				
1 intervals:				Taper
RUN x 1 steady:	RUN, 1 steady	ROW x 2 threshold	ROW x 2 threshold	ROW 1 x 1500 ints:
WEIGHTS x 1 power	ROW x 2 threshold	3000: 1 x 1500 ints:	3000: 1 x 1500 ints:	1 hills, others steady
ROW x 1 power,	3000: 1 x 1500 ints:	1 x 1000 ints,.	1 x 1000 ints,.	2 x 1000 ints,.
1 overspeed, 1 time	1 x 1000 ints,.	CIRCUITS x 2	CIRCUITS x 1	
trial, 1 short ints.	WEIGHTS x 2 power			INDOOR ROW
CIRCUITS x 2	CIRCUITS x 2			CHAMPIONSHIPS

Figure 20.9 In his last mesocycle, the athlete has one major mountain bike competition; again this is a two-day event and is followed just two weeks later by a mountain marathon, also a two-day event. In the final few weeks of this mesocycle he cuts right back on cross training in an attempt to peak for the British Indoor Rowing Championships, in which he took 51st place, completing 2000 metres in 6:28:6.

Heptathlon	Decathlon
• 100 m hurdles	• 100 m sprint
• High jump	• Long jump
• Shot put	• Shot put
• 200 m sprint	• High jump
• Long jump	• 400 m sprint
• Javelin	• 110 m hurdles
• 800 m	• Discus
	• Pole vault
	• Javelin
	• 1500 m

The modern, or military pentathlon is based on the skills needed by a battlefield courier, and was first included in the Olympic Games of 1912. From 1952 to 1992 it was a team event. Modern pentathlon is a five-day contest involving five events:

- an equestrian steeplechase over a distance of about 450 m;

- a series of épée fencing matches;

- pistol shooting at standing silhouette targets;

- 300-metre freestyle swim;

- 4,000-metre cross-country run.

Scoring is on a point basis, the individual and team winners being decided by total scores from the five events.

Triathlon and modern pentathlon are multi-sport, rather than multidiscipline, events. Traditionally encompassing swimming, road bike and road running triathlons now often encompass mountain bike, cross-country or fell running and rowing or kayaking. Similarly and growing from the challenge of triathlon, there is a huge increase in the popularity of adventure sports. The events are drawn from rock climbing, horse riding, cycling or mountain biking, fell running, kayaking or canoeing and mountaineering. Most often they are team events, the whole team having to complete the whole course, which tests the skill and fitness of the individuals in the team and the ability of the team to work together.

Adventure racing

Adventure racing is set to return to New Zealand in November with the announcement today that Wanaka is to be the host for the opening venue for this year's Southern Traverse.

As in previous years the location of the race course is still kept a secret until the night before the race but in the announcement today the organisers confirmed that there will be 3 mountain passes, 2 paddling sections, 3 mountain biking sections, and a huge (175m + 75m) abseiling section.

The race is due to start on Monday the 10th November and it is expected that the first competitors will reach the finish line in Queenstown after 4 days and some 350kms of racing.

Taken from Southern Traverse media release, 22nd Oct 1997, 'Wanaka announced as the Opening Venue for the 1997 Southern Traverse'

Training for multi-sport challenges

For the multi-sport athlete the challenge is to combine skill with fitness training to meet the demands of all the disciplines or events involved in the sport. This demands that multi-sport training is used wisely in order to get maximum benefits.

To write a multi-sport training programme for multidiscipline sports a long-term approach must be taken. The first need is to identify the top priority event.

For instance for a triathlete who is pretty reasonable at swimming, cycling and running, top priority may become cycling as this covers the furthest distance and so has the potential to make up the most time; however, for someone who is a poor swimmer, swimming may become priority as they may be losing too much time on this event.

Whatever training is included has to fit into general life. Athletes with the ability to devote their life to training are rare, especially in events that don't attract large sponsorship and prize money; so lifestyle restraints, such as working hours and free time, family responsibilities etc., may limit the time available to devote to training. It is therefore all the more important to ensure that the training programme is designed well.

Macrocycle					
January	February	March	April	May	June
5 12 19 26	2 9 16 23	2 9 16 23 30	6 13 20 27	4 11 18 25	1 8 15 22 29

Mesocycles			
05-Jan	16-Feb	06-Apr	11-May
Base 1 increase strength esp upper body	base 2 increase upper body strength increase muscular endurance	Build up Power and endurance	specificity specificity and taper
Strength – total body build up distance run and cycle Training at 80 to 100% VO2 max, some intervals of 2 mins work 2 mins rest	Start canoeing. increase upper body strength increase cyling and running distance. Longer distance at 70 to 90% VO2 max. Increase running/ cycling/canoeing time to 90 to 120 minutes.	power weights, hill training running and cycling. Long weekend training sessions Lots of long slow distance with some high intensity.	hill cycling and intervals run hills off road two week taper, decrease frequency and time keep intensity high.

Figure 20.10 *The adventure athlete whose programme is illustrated here is competing in a race that involves canoeing, cycling, and fell running. Her first two mesocycles aim to improve strength and endurance, then she will add power, and finally train specifically for the event*

Part IV
Useful resources

21 Useful stretches

Calf stretch

Stand with one leg forwards and bent at the knee, the other leg back with knee straight, keep the heel of the rear foot on the floor and lean forwards. You will feel the stretch in the back of the lower leg. Make sure your back foot is pointing forwards.

Repeat with the other leg.

Lower-calf stretch

As above, but bend the back knee until you feel the stretch move lower down in the calf muscle.

Thigh stretch

Stand on one leg and make sure not to arch the lower back; take hold of the ankle of the other foot and pull your heel towards your buttocks. Keep your knees together and push the pubic bone forwards. You will feel the stretch at the front of the thigh. It helps to relax into this stretch if you hold onto a wall or another person for balance.

Hamstring stretch

Stand with one leg forwards and one leg back; keep the front leg straight and bend the back leg, which is taking your weight.

Place your hands on your bent back leg for support and lean forwards until the stretch is felt in back of the leg above the knee. Repeat the stretch with the other leg.

Side stretch

Stand with your knees slightly bent and keep your hips fixed centrally between your feet. Reach over your head with one hand, supporting your body weight by putting the other hand on your hip. Reach upwards first to feel a mild stretch in the side of the body and as this eases reach over the head to bend the body sideways and increase the stretch.

Chest stretch

Stand with your knees slightly bent. Place one hand flat against a wall and turn the shoulder forwards. You will feel the stretch on the front of the shoulder and across the chest. Repeat on the other side.

Seated hamstring stretch

Sit with one leg straight forwards and your toes pointing upwards, and the other leg out to the side in a comfortable position. Lean forwards from the hips, keeping your head up. You will feel the stretch at the back of the straight leg. Repeat the stretch with the other leg.

Inner thigh stretch

Sit upright with the soles of your feet together. Press your knees slowly towards the floor. You will feel the stretch in your inner thigh.

Back stretch

Sit on the floor with your legs crossed and lean forwards, letting your chin drop to your chest. You will feel the stretch in whichever part of your back is tightest.

Where you feel a stretch will depend on your flexibility and which muscles are tightest, as well as on the activities you have been doing. There are very many different stretches and the reader is recommended to get a book on stretching, as different stretches suit different individuals.

1RM one repetition maximum: the resistance needed to limit the lifter to one repetition only. A second repetition of the exercise cannot be achieved.

Actin filaments see **myofilaments**.

Active lifestyle A lifestyle incorporating physical activity integrated into daily life. Physical activity includes walking or cycling to the shops instead of using the car, walking upstairs instead of taking the elevator, climbing onto chairs or steps to reach things in high cupboards or reaching down for things in low cupboards rather than storing things within easy reach, etc.

Active living As defined by Fitness Canada 1991, is 'a way of life in which physical activity is valued and integrated into daily life'.

Active range of movement The range of movement where only the muscles affecting that movement are used.

Acute Having a rapid onset and short duration.

Adenosine di-phosphate (ADP) When the high-energy bond in adenosine tri-phosphate (ATP) is broken, adenosine di-phosphate and one free phosphate molecule result.

Adenosine tri-phosphate (ATP) Made up of one molecule of adenosine and three phosphate molecules attached by high-energy bonds. Energy is trapped inside these bonds.

Aerobic power (VO$_2$max) The maximum amount of oxygen that can be extracted from the air and utilised in the working muscles for the aerobic production of energy.

Agonist Muscles work in pairs. The muscle contracting to affect the movement is called the agonist. The muscle opposite that, which has to relax in order for movement to happen, is called the antagonist.

Alveolar Small airsacs in the lungs, the site of pulmonary gaseous exchange.

Anabolism The building up of muscle tissue; the constructive phase of metabolism.

Anaerobic glycolysis The utilisation of carbohydrate, which is stored in the body as glycogen and can be converted into glucose and thence into a substance called pyruvate.

Anaerobic threshold Also called onset of blood lactate accumulation (OBLA) or lactate threshold. The workload at which lactate production is greater than its removal and so lactate builds up to a level where muscular contraction is interfered with.

Antagonist Muscles work in pairs. The muscle contracting to affect the movement is called the agonist. The muscle opposite that, which has to relax in order for movement to happen, is called the antagonist.

Arteries carry blood away from the heart.

Audax The long-distance cycling club see p. 39

Biomechanics An application of the principles of mechanics to human or animal movement.

Biopsies Muscle biopsy is a procedure whereby a needle with a canula is inserted into the muscle tissue and a small piece of muscle tissue is withdrawn.

Blood lipids Fats such as triglicerides, high-density lipoproteins (HDL), low-density lipoproteins (LDL) and very low-density lipoproteins (VLDL), circulating in the blood plasma.

Blood plasma The fluid portion of the blood.

Bronchial tubes Tubular airways leading into the alveolar of the lungs.

Capillaries Small blood vessels forming a network throughout the body.

Cardiac drift or **Heart rate drift** With the onset of exercise, the heart rate increases from resting levels and stabilises, usually changing very little during 5–10 minutes of steady state exercise. However, if exercise continues for a longer period of time, the heart rate continues to rise and is accompanied by a decrease in stroke volume.

Cardiac muscle The muscle of the heart.

Cardiac output The volume of blood pumped out by the heart per minute, measured by the stroke volume times the heart rate.

Cardiovascular fitness A level of aerobic exercise that taxes the cardiovascular system enough to stimulate physiological adaptation, such that it is able to deliver and utilise oxygen sufficiently to fuel prolonged intensive exercise.

Cardiovascular training (CV) The improvement of the efficiency of the heart.

Catabolism The breaking down of muscle tissue; the destructive phase of metabolism.

Cholesterol A fat that is ingested in the diet and also produced in the liver. Foods high in cholesterol are derived from animal sources. High levels of cholesterol and especially a high ratio of total cholesterol to high-density lipoproteins is associated with increased risk of atherosclerosis and coronary heart disease.

Chronic Of gradual onset or long duration.

Circuit training A series of exercises arranged in such a manner that they are each performed for a period of time or a number of repetitions in sequence, in order to constitute a complete workout.

COH Chemical symbol for carbohydrate.

Competition Competition phase, within which the competition or series of competitions take place. The athlete must peak and retain form.

Concentration gradient Gases diffuse from high to low concentration along a concentration gradient.

Concentric During a concentric contraction the two ends of the muscle move closer together and the muscle shortens.

Conditioning Conditioning whereby elements of fitness such as strength and endurance are trained.

Contra-indicated exercise An exercise that is not recommended for a particular individual because of previous injury, present medical condition or his or her particular biomechanics.

Coronary heart disease (CHD) A disease of the coronary arteries, i.e. those supplying the heart, in which they become narrow and in the worst cases completely occluded. If a primary artery is occluded and no alternative route is available, that part of the myocardium normally supplied by that artery cannot function and a myocardial infarction, or heart attack, occurs. Characteristics known to increase the probability of developing coronary heart disease include cigarette smoking, elevated blood lipids (LDL to HDL ratio), inactivity, hypertension, family history of heart disease, psychological stress and obesity.

Creatine phosphate A product of protein metabolism stored in the muscles, which can be broken down to release energy. It is very responsive to the muscle's needs and is capable of supplying energy very quickly but only for an extremely short period of time.

Diastole The resting phase or relaxation of cardiac muscle that allows the heart to refill with blood and allows coronary circulation to occur.

Diastolic The blood pressure measurement during the phase of diastole.

Eccentric When a muscle is generating force in an attempt to overcome a resistance but is in fact lengthening (giving in to the resistance), it is working in the eccentric phase of the contraction.

Efferent nerves Motor nerves that transmit messages from the central nervous system to the body.

Endurance The ability of a muscle or group of muscles to overcome a resistance for an extended period of time, that is, more than once. The ability to bear a physical workload for extended periods of time.

Enzyme A complex protein formed in living cells and assisting chemical processes without being changed itself, i.e. organic catalysts.

Ergometer a piece of equipment that is calibrated and produces measurable units of work enabling a person's work output to be measured.

Estimated maximum heart rate An estimation of maximum heart rate based on a person's age. The most used formula is 220 minus age = maximum heart rate. As this is an estimation it is not accurate, but is used as a safe way of estimating workload.

Fast glycolytic fibres (FG) Muscle fibres otherwise known as type II, well adapted for anaerobic respiration, and reaching peak tension very quickly.

Fast oxidative glycolytic (FOG) Type IIA muscle fibres that are similar to fast glycolytic fibres that with training are capable of adapting to aerobic respiration.

FITT Frequency, intensity, time (volume) and type of exercise; can be manipulated to form a training programme specific to the athlete's needs.

Fixator muscles Muscles that check unwanted movement in a joint or joint complex.

Force Impetus that causes an object to be formed or moved.

Forced vital capacity The amount of air that can be forced out of the lungs in one breath.

Glycogen The form in which carbohydrate is stored in the body.

Golgi Tendon Organs (GTOs) Nerve receptors located within the tendons. Tension on a tendon, as may happen during stretch but more often occurs during a muscle contraction, may fire the Golgi tendon organ reflex, causing the muscle to relax.

H_2O Chemical symbol for water.

Haemoglobin The iron-containing pigment of red blood cells that carries oxygen in the blood.

HDL to LDL ratio The ratio of high-density lipoproteins to low-density lipoproteins found circulating in the blood. A high proportion of high-density lipoproteins is associated with a reduced risk of developing atheroma.

High-density lipoprotein (HDL) Lipoprotein contained in blood plasma and composed of a high proportion of protein and a low proportion of triglyceride and cholesterol. A high concentration of HDL is associated with lowered risk of coronary heart disease.

Hormones Chemical messengers produced by the body and transported in the blood to its target tissue.

Hyperextension The over-extension of a joint.

Hyperplasia The theory of hyperplasia states that the muscle fibres themselves split, creating extra muscle fibres within a single muscle.

Hypertension Raised blood pressure. If resting values are greater than 140 mm/90mm Hg chronic hypertension exists.

Hypertrophy The theory of hypertrophy is that muscle filaments increase in number within each single muscle fibre, thus increasing the cross-sectional area of each muscle fibre.

Insulin A hormone produced by the pancreas, used in carbohydrate metabolism and transportation of glucose to the working muscles.

Insulin response The production of insulin in response to ingestion of carbohydrate. As the body becomes more sensitive to insulin, less is produced by the pancreas.

Insulin sensitivity The taking-up of glucose from the blood by the working muscles and the fat cells in response to output of insulin by the pancreas. As the body becomes fitter the response to insulin becomes mores sensitive.

Interval training Consists of intermittent exercise with regular rest periods between the work periods. The ratio of work to rest is manipulated according to the desired training effect.

Isokinetic contraction A muscle contraction in which the speed of movement around a joint is controlled by an external force.

Isometric contraction A muscle contraction force is created but no movement across the joint occurs.

Isotonic contraction A muscle contraction in which there is movement around a joint.

Karvonen formula MHR − RHR × *% + RHR = *% of VO_2max, where MHR = max heart rate and RHR = resting heart rate,
e.g. 185 − 54 × 75% + 54 = 152. MHR - RHR × *% + RHR = heart rate at 75% MHRR.

Lactate A product of anaerobic metabolism that builds up in the form of lactic acid.

Lactate threshold Also called anaerobic threshold, or onset of blood lactate accumulation (OBLA). The workload at which lactate production is greater than lactate removal and so lactate builds up to a level such that muscular contraction is interfered with.

Lactate tolerance The body's ability to tolerate lactate build up.

Lactic acid Lactate that builds up in the muscle thereby blocking muscle contraction, causing a burning sensation and forcing the body to slow down or stop when the intensity of exercise is too high for too long a period of time.

Low-density Lipoprotein (LDL) Lipoprotein contained in blood plasma and composed of a moderate proportion of protein with a high proportion of cholesterol. A high concentration of LDL is associated with an increased risk of coronary heart disease.

Macrocycle The period of time from now until you reach your main goal.

Maximum heart rate or **Peak heart rate** maximum heart rate possible for an individual during any given exercise modality.

Maximum heart rate reserve (MHRR) True maximum heart rate minus true resting heart rate.

Maximum oxygen uptake or **VO$_2$max** The highest amount of oxygen that the body can consume for the aerobic production of ATP. That is the amount of oxygen that the body can take in and utilise in the working muscles for the production of energy.

Mesocycles You can split the macrocycle up into shorter sections during which you focus on particular elements of training. These shorter sections or phases are called mesocycles.

Metabolic enzyme profile Muscle fibres can be characterised by distinguishing the enzymes characteristic of the different energy systems that they use.

Mitochondria The sites within the muscle cell where aerobic metabolism, that is the oxidation of fats and carbohydrate, takes place.

mM = mMols A measure of blood lactate measured in mMol's per litre. Anaerobic threshold is normally said to be at 4.0 mM/l

Motor end plate The interface between the nerve ending and the muscle cell is known as the motor end plate.

Motor unit Each nerve ending serves a number of muscle fibres. The nerve ending and its associated muscle fibres are known collectively as a single motor unit.

Multi gym Resistance equipment using systems of levers and pulleys and weight stacks.

Muscular Endurance The ability of a muscle or group of muscles to exert force to overcome a resistance but for an extended period of time. It is an expression of the ability to repeatedly generate muscular force.

Muscular Strength An expression of the amount of force generated by one single maximum contraction. It refers to the ability of a muscle or group of muscles to exert maximum force to overcome a resistance.

Myocardium The muscular wall of the heart.

Myofilaments These are tiny filaments of proteins called actin and myosin. When a muscle fibre is innervated to contract, these actin and myosin filaments slide across each other causing the muscle to contract. This is known as the sliding filament theory.

Myogenic Changes These changes involve an increase in the density or the size of the muscle.

Myoglobin A pigment found in muscle that transports oxygen from the cell membrane to the mitochondria.

Myosin filaments see **myofilaments**.

Neurogenic Changes Changes happening at a neurogenic level, that is within the nerve pathways.

Norms The average or mean measurement taken from a population.

Obesity A condition in which a person's body fat percentage is above that which increases disease risk. Medical opinion is divided over the actual body fat percentages classified as constituting a condition of obesity.

OBLA onset of blood lactate

accumulation - also called anaerobic threshold, or lactate threshold. The workload at which lactate production is greater than lactate removal and so lactate builds up to a level such that muscular contraction is interfered with.

Occluded Completely blocked.

Olympic Weight Lifting strength sport Consisting of the combined score from two free weight lifts. The Clean and Jerk and the Snatch.

Osteoporosis A disease affecting bone density and strength which is reduced such that fractures occur spontaneously or with minor falls and bumps. Sometimes known as brittle bone disease, osteoporosis affects one in four women in Britain by the age of 60 years and this becomes one in two by the age of 70 years. Although this disease mainly affects women due to the loss of the hormone oestrogen after the menopause, the number of men also affected is growing.

Overload The body only adapts to unaccustomed demand. To improve you must ask it to do more than it is used to doing.

Oxidative Enzymes are the enzymes involved in aerobic metabolism.

Partial pressure The pressure exerted by individual gases in a mixture of gases

Passive range of movement Demonstrated when joint movement is assisted by an outside force.

Peak heart rate Maximum heart rate possible for an individual during any given exercise modality.

Periodisation A method of structuring training in order to prevent overtraining and optimise peak performance.

Periosteum The connective tissue sheath wrapped around bone.

Peripheral Neuromuscular Facilitation (PNF) Stretching utilising the Golgi Tendon Organs (GTO) reflex by purposely putting the tendon under tension thus causing the reflex action of muscle relaxation.

Power The product of force and velocity, or strength x speed. Power is a product of the speed of contraction and force of contraction with peak power output generally occurring at around 30% of maximum velocity.

Proprioreceptive Sensory information produced by sensory nerve cells which detect the position of the body and its parts, extent and force of movement, muscular tension and physical pressure.

Pyruvate Carbohydrate is broken down into pyruvate which is further broken down, to release energy.

R.I.C.E. Rest, Ice, Compression, Elevation. A formula for effective first aid in the case of closed soft tissue injuries. In order to reduce swelling, the limb should be rested, ice should be applied, some form of compression should be applied and the limb should be elevated.

Rate of Perceived Exertion RPE Scale rates the intensity of exercise by how the exercise feels e.g. somewhat hard, easy, very hard.

Reciprocal innervation Any movement involves contracting individual muscle fibres or groups of muscle fibres in the right sequence to cause that movement to happen. Simultaneously opposing muscle fibres must be allowed to relax in order that they do not block that movement from happening.

Repetitions Numbers of times of repeating an exercise .

Repetitions maximum or **RM** The greatest resistance that you can overcome for a particular lift. Thus the heaviest weight that can be lifted for 10 repetitions (i.e. an eleventh is not possible) is known as 10 repetitions maximum (10 reps max or 10RM). The heaviest weight that can be lifted for 6 repetitions is known as 6RM. The maximum for one repetition would be 1RM.

Resting heart rate (RHR) Taken in the morning, after waking up (gently), emptying the bladder and then resting again for a few minutes to allow the heart rate to settle.

SAID principle SAID stands for Specific Adaptation to Imposed Demand.

Slow Oxidative fibres (SO) May be termed Type I fibres. They have a lot of mitochondria and oxidative enzymes and a plentiful supply of capillaries. They are well adapted for aerobic respiration.

Smooth muscle Found in the gastro intestinal tract.

Steady state Occurs when nearly all the cost of the exercise is met by aerobic metabolism.

Strength The ability of a muscle or group of muscles to overcome a resistance once.

Striated or Skeletal muscle The muscle which is attached to the skeletal system and is under voluntary control. This is the muscle that we use to maintain posture and affect movement. This is also the muscle that is of importance in relation to fitness and specifically in relation to muscular strength, muscular endurance and power.

Stroke volume The amount of blood ejected from the left ventricle of the heart during contraction.

Systole The active phase or contraction of cardiac muscle to expel blood from the heart chambers.

Systolic Measurement of blood pressure taken during systole

Taper Reduction in training levels to ensure an athlete is fresh for a competitive event.

Tendons The connective tissue that attach muscles to bone.

Tidal volume The amount of air that is moved in or out of the lungs in one breath.

Type I fibres May be termed Slow Oxidative fibres (SO). They have a lot of mitochondria and oxidative enzymes and a plentiful supply of capillaries. They are well adapted for aerobic respiration.

Type IIB fibres May be termed Fast Glycolytic fibres (FG). They are well adapted for anaerobic respiration, and they reach peak tension very quickly.

Type IIA fibres Fast Oxidative Glycolytic (FOG) fibres are similar to Fast Glycolytic fibres but with training are capable of adapting to aerobic respiration.

Veins Carry blood towards the heart.

Vertebrae Are the individual bones that make up the spine.

BIBLIOGRAPHY

Survival of the Fittest
   Mike Stroud
   Jonathan Cape, London

Running For Fitness
   Owen Barder
   A&C Black, London

The Complete Guide to Endurance Training
   Jon Ackland
   A&C Black, London

The Complete Guide to Strength Training
   Anita Bean
   A&C Black, London

The Complete Guide To Sports Nutrition
   (2nd edition)
   Anita Bean
   A&C, Black London

Flexibility For Sport
   Bob Smith
   Crowood Press

Fitness Programming
   Fiona Hayes
   Summit Directions Ltd.

Physiology of Fitness
   Brian J Sharkey
   Human Kinetics

Serious Training for Serious Athletes
   Rob Sleamaker
   Leisure Press

Swimming For Fitness
   Kelvin Juba
   A&C Black, London

Chapter 1

1   IHRSA

2   Claude Bouchard, 'Discussion: hereditary fitness and health', in Bouchard et al. (eds.), *Exercise, Fitness and Health: A Consensus of Current Knowledge* Human Kinetics

3   S.J. Jacobs and B.L Berson, 'Injuries to runners: A study of entrants to a 10,000 metre race', *American Journal of Sports Medicine*, 14 (1986), 151–155

4   S.N. Blair, H.W. Kohl and N.N. Goodyear, 'Rates and risks for running and exercise injuries: Studies in three populations', *Res. Q. Exerc. Sport*, 58 (1987), 221–228

5   J.G. Garrick, D.M. Gillian and P. Whiteside, 'The epidemiology of aerobic dance injuries', *American Journal of Sports Medicine*, 14 (1986)P, 67–72

6   The Osteoporosis Association

7   American College of Sports Medicine, 'Position Stand on the Recommended Quantity and Quality of Exercise for Developing and Maintaining Cardiorespiratory and Muscular Fitness, and Flexibility in Healthy Adults', *Medicine and Science in Sport and Exercise*, 30/6 (June 1988)

8   *Physical Activity and Health, A Report of the Surgeon General*, US Department of Health and Human Services, Centers for Disease Control and Prevention, National Center for Chronic Disease Prevention and Health Promotion (Atlanta, Ga., 1996)

Chapter 2

1   Taken from the Southern Traverse website at http://www.southerntraverse.com

2   E.L. Melanson, P.S. Freedson and S. Jungbluth, 'Changes in VO$_2$max and maximal treadmill time after nine weeks of running or in-line skate training', *Medicine and Science in Sport and Exercise*, 28/11 (1996), 1422–1426

3   D.L. Mutton, S.F. Loy, D.M. Rogers, J.G. Holland, W.J. Vincent and M. Heng, 'Effect of run vs. combined cycle/run training on VO$_2$max and running performance', *Medicine and Science in Sport and Exercise*, 25/12 (1993), 1393–1397

4   H. Tanaka, 'Effect of cross-training. Transfer of training effects on VO$_2$max between cycling, running and swimming', *Sports Med.* 18/5 (Nov. 1994), 330–339

5   M.C. Gaiga and D. Docherty, 'The effect of an aerobic interval training programme on intermittent anaerobic performance', *Canadian Journal of Applied Physiology*, 20/4 (1995), 452–464

6   R.E. Johnston, T.J. Quinn, R. Kertzer and N.B. Vroman, 'Strength training in

female distance runners: Impact on running economy', *Medicine and Science in Sport and Exercise*, 27/5 suppl. (1995)

[7] D.L. Blessing, B.L. Gravelle, Y.T. Wang, and K.C. Kim, 'The influence of co-activation on the adaptive response to concurrent strength and endurance training in women', ibid.

[8] McCarthy et al., 'Compatibility of adaptive responses with combining strength and endurance training', *Medicine and Science in Sport and Exercise*, 27/3 (1995), 429–436

Chapter 5

[1] Steven E. Robbins and Gerard J. Gouw, 'Athletic footwear: Unsafe due to perceptual illusions', *Medicine and Science in Sport and Exercise*, 23/2 (1991), 217–224

Chapter 8

[1] C. Bouchard, 'Overview of the Consensus Symposium', *Toward Active Living* Human Kinetics

Chapter 9

[1] D.C. Kernie, S. Dinan and A. Young, 'Health promotion and physical activity', in *Textbook of Geriatric Medicine and Gerontology*, 5th edition (in press)

[2] S.D.R. Harridge and A.Young, 'Skeletal muscle', in M.S.J. Pathy (ed.), *Principles and Practice of Geriatric Medicine* (London: John Wiley, 1997)

[3] D.I. Levi, A. Young, D.A. Skelton and A.-L. Yeo, 'Strength, power and functional ability', in M. Passeri (ed.), *Geriatrics* (Rome: Edizioni Internazionali, 1994), 85–93. A. Young, 'Exercise physiology in geriatric practice', *Acta Med. Scand.* Suppl. 711 (1986), 227–232

Chapter 10

[1] W. Evans and I. Rosenburg, *Biomarkers* (New York: Simon & Schuster, 1992)

[2] A. Young. 'Strength and power', in J.G. Evans and T.F. Williams (eds.), *Oxford Textbook of Geriatric Medicine* (Oxford: Oxford University Press, 1992), 597–601. C.T.M. Davies, D.O. Thomas and M.J. White, 'Mechanical properties of young and elderly human muscle'. *Acta Med. Scand.* Suppl. 711 (1986), 219–226

[3] I. Hardy, 'Improving active range of hip flexion', *Res. Q. Exerc. Sport* (USA) 56/2 (1985), 111–114

Chapter 11

[1] Ronald Maughan, 'Nutrition', Gatorade Sports Science Exchange, 4/4 (1993)

[2] J. Wilmore and D. Costill, 'Physiology of sport and exercise', *Human Kinetics* (1994), 363–365

[3] L.E. Armstrong, D.L. Costill and W.J. Fink, 'Influence of diuretic-induced dehydration on competitive running performance', *Medicine and Science in Sport and Exercise*, 17 (1985), 456–461

[4] American College of Sports Medicine, 'Position stand on exercise and fluid replacement', *Medicine and Science in Sport and Exercise*, 28 (1996), pp. i–vii

[5] D.L. Costill and K.E. Sparks, 'Rapid fluid replacement following thermal dehydration', *Journal of Applied Physiology*, 34 (1973), 299–303

[6] Bob Murray, 'Fluid Replacement: The American College of Sports Medicine Position Stand', *Gatorade Sports Science Exchange*, 63/9 suppl. 4 (1996)

Chapter 12

[1] J. Wilmore and D. Costill, 'Physiology of sport and exercise', *Human Kinetics* (1994), 217

[2] Per Olaf Astrand and Kaare Rodahl, *Textbook of Work Physiology*, 3rd edition (New York: McGraw Hill), 310

[3] J.K. Kalis, B.J. Freund, M.J. Joyner, S.M. Jilka, J. Nittolo and J.H. Wilmore, 'Effect of beta-block on the drift in O2 consumption during prolonged exercise', *Journal of Applied Physiology* (USA), 64/2 (1988), 753–758

[4] R.L. Terjung, 'Muscle adaptations to aerobic training', *Gatorade Sports Science Exchange*, 54

Chapter 13

[1] Per Olaf Astrand and Kaare Rodahl, *Textbook of Work Physiology*, 3rd edition (New York: McGraw Hill), 333

Chapter 14

[1] Miriam E. Nelson, *Strong Women Stay Young* (Bantam Books, 1997)

[2] M.H. Stone, S.J. Fleck, N.T. Triplett and W.J. Kraemer, 'The health and performance related potential of resistance training', *Sports Medicine*, 11/4 (19??)

[3] Allied Dunbar National Fitness Survey Report (April 1992)

[4] *Physical Activity and Health, A Report of the Surgeon General*, US Department of Health and Human Services, Centers for Disease Control and Prevention, National Center for Chronic Disease Prevention and Health Promotion (Atlanta, Ga., 1996)

[5] L. Barton, H.A. Bird, M. Lindsay, J. Newton and V. Wright 'The effect of different joint interventions on the range of movement at a joint', *Journal of Orthopaedic Rheumatology* (UK), 8/2 (1995), 87 92

[6] P.D. Gollnick and B. Saltin, 'Significance of skeletal muscle oxidative enzyme enhancement with endurance training', *Clinical Physiology* (UK), 2/1 (1982), 1–12. L.S. Sidossis, C.A. Stuart, G.I. Shulman, G.D. Lopaschuk and R.R. Wolfe, 'Glucose plus insulin regulate fat oxidation by controlling the rate of fatty acid entry into the

mitochondria', *Journal of Clinical Investigation* (USA), 98/10 (1996). P.J. Abernethy, R. Thayer and A.W. Taylor, 'Acute and chronic responses of skeletal muscle to endurance and sprint exercise. A review', *Sports Medicine* (NZ), 10/6 (1990), 365–389

[7] P.L. Greenhaff, 'Creatine: Its role in physical performance and fatigue and its application as a sports food supplement', *Insider* 3/1 (March 1995). B. Dawson, M. Cutler, A. Moody, S. Lawrence, C. Goodman and N. Randall, 'Effects of oral creatine loading on single and repeated maximal short sprints', *Australian Journal of Science and Medicine in Sport*, 27/3 (1995)

[8] L.H. Boobis, Williams and Wooton, 'Human muscle metabolism during brief maximal exercise', *Journal of Applied Physiology*, 338 (1982), 21–22

[9] G.C. Bogdanis, M.E. Nevill, L.H. Boobis and H.K.A. Lakomy, 'Contribution of phosphocreatine and aerobic metabolism to energy supply during repeated sprint exercise', *Journal of Applied Physiology* (USA), 80/3 (1996)

[10] R.E. Johnston, T.J. Quinn, R. Kertzer, and N.B. Vroman, 'Strength training in female distance runners: Impact on running economy'. D.L. Blessing, B.L. Gravelle, Y.T. Wang and C.K. Kim, 'The influence of co-activation on the adaptive response to concurrent strength and endurance training in women', and B. Gravelle and D.L. Blessing, 'Physiological adaptation in women concurrently training for strength and endurance', *Medicine and Science in Sport and Exercise*, 27/5, suppl. abstr. 47 (1995). T. Hortobagyi, F.I. Katch and P.F. Lachance, 'Effects of simultaneous training for strength and endurance on upper and lower body strength and running performance', *The Journal of Sports Medicine and Physical Fitness*, 31 (1991), 20–30

[11] J.D. McDougall, D.G. Sale, J.R. Moroz, G.C.B. Elder, J.R. Sutton and H. Howard, 'Mitochondrial volume density in human skeletal muscle following heavy resistance training', *Medicine and Science in Sports*, 11 (1979), 164–166

Chapter 15

[1] Claude Bouchard, 'Discussion: Hereditary fitness and health', in Bouchard *et al.* (eds.), Exercise, *Fitness and Health: A Consensus of Current Knowledge* Human Kinetics

Chapter 18

[1] I. Astrand, P.-O. Astrand, E.H. Christiansen and R. Hedman, 'Intermittent Muscular Work', *Acta Physio. Scand.* 48 (1960), 443. I. Astrand, P.-O. Astrand, E.H. Christiansen and R. Hedman, 'Myohaemoglobin as an oxygen store in man', ibid. 454

[2] L. Gullstrand, 'Physiological responses to short duration high intensity rowing', *Canadian Journal of Applied Physiology*, 21/3 (1996), 197–208

Chapter 20

[1] E.G. McFarland and M. Wasik, 'Injuries in female collegiate swimmers due to swimming and cross training', *Clinical Journal of Sport Medicine* (USA), 6/3 (1996)

[2] B. Ruby, R. Robergs, G. Leadbetter, C. Mermier, T. Chick and D. Stark, 'Cross-training between cycling and running in untrained females', *Journal of Sports Medicine and Physical Fitness* (Italy), 36/4 (1996)

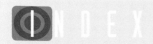